W9-CYS-540

PAN

Artesia, CA.

YOUR

Your Complete Personal Guide

HEALTH

To Wellness

YOUR

Nutrition & Disease Prevention

CHOICE

YOUR

Your Complete Personal Guide

HEALTH

To Wellness

YOUR

Nutrition & Disease Prevention

CHOICE

by
DR. M. TED MORTER. JR.

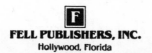

FELL PUBLISHERS, INC.
Hollywood, Florida

Library of Congress Cataloging-in-Publication Data

Morter, M. T.
    Your health, your choice : your complete personal guide to
wellness, nutrition & disease prevention / by M. Ted Morter, Jr. —
1st ed.
        p.   cm.
    ISBN 0-8119-0655-8 (cloth) : $17.95. — ISBN 0-8119-0667-1 (paper)
$12.95
    1. Nutrition.   I. Title.
RA784.M628   1990
613.2–dc20   90-13801
                                                                CIP

Manufactured in the United States of America
AGF-PA
10 9 8 7 6 5 4 3 2 1

To my wife Marjorie, without whose encouragement, patience, and tolerance of the turbulence I caused in her life during its gestation period this book would not have been written, and to the many patients who prodded me to write it.

Contents

Tables, Charts, and Lists

Foreword

While it is axiomatic that a well body needs no treatment, few of us are completely well. The most common cause of "unwellness" is diet. More specifically, the real cause of our lack of wellness is the "recommended" diet advocated by most nutritionists of today.

There is no doubt about the efficacy of the "standard American diet." As our western dietary customs spread throughout the world, our western "unwellness" spreads also. The cardiovascular problems of the people of Scandinavia, Japan, and other areas and countries are increasing to a point that rivals our own. Other health problems, such as increased bacterial and viral diseases, have also increased as our high-fat and high-protein diet spreads. Efficacy of diet then becomes causality: diet is more than effective for health; it can cause wellness or unwellness. High stress, high fat intake, high life, and high protein foods all contribute to our "unwellness."

Dr. Morter deals well with the subject of unwellness. At first glance, the premises he advocates may seem unorthodox. However, as his explanations progress throughout the book, his entire treatise becomes captivating. The ideas presented are simple and easy to accept. *Your Health, Your Choice* does a commendable job of simplifying the very difficult concept that the body has an innate ability to keep itself in tune via "proper" nutrition. We may, in this book, finally have a health-choice definition for the word "proper" in regard to nutrition. Well done, Dr. Morter.

Robert L. Brown, Ph.D.
Nutrition and Biochemistry
Dallas, Texas
April 1990

Acknowledgements

Writing a book of this nature cannot be accomplished single-handedly. The material has evolved through association with other doctors and with patients. Hundreds of doctors and patients have served as sources of inspiration, information, and encouragement. In particular, John M. Clark, D.C., and the other doctors at Morter Chiropractic Clinic have contributed their observations and expertise as I developed the concepts in this book. Other members of my clinic staff, the doctors who attend my seminars, and their patients over the years have provided support and assistance in the research and preparation of background information.

Many people outside of the clinic have also been of inestimable help and encouragement: Robert L. Brown, Ph.D., my technical advisor, who contributed his time, efforts, and the Foreword to this book; Stanley Plagenhoef, Ph.D.; Richard Knight, M.D.; Charles E. Wiley, M.D.; Glen Bounds, Ph.D.; and Peg Blackadar, R.N., offered generous endorsements that appear on the cover. Others who have contributed insightful suggestions include Anne Inman, Steve Hinkey, D.C., Tom Hecox, Sandra Tindall, Jean Waterman, and Dick Whiteside.

On the production side, to Don Lessne, my publisher, goes the perseverance award for his relentless pursuit and capture of just the right title; to Allan Taber my appreciation for his valuable editing advice; and acknowledgement to Pat Kelly who wrote the text.

A special loving thanks to my family. Each of them has been not only supportive and encouraging but has gracefully withstood the tumult that sometimes accompanies a project of this size. Sons, Dr. Ted Morter, III, and Dr. Tom Morter, and daughter, Dr. Sue Morter, have offered valuable suggestions and loving criticism when necessary. Most especially, though, my thanks go to my wife, Marjorie. She is my behind-the-scenes support, counsel, and best friend who, for over 30 years, has made my life particularly satisfying.

Inside These Pages You'll Find That...

Not everyone who is sick feels bad...

Living shouldn't be an exercise in progressive deterioration...

You don't have to be sick...

Age is no excuse for disease or aches and pains...

How well your body functions depends on what you give it to work with...

Medicines may save your life, but they can't heal...

Only your body can heal itself...

You can evaluate your health before symptoms of disease appear...

If you have to increase the potency or dosage of your medicine to get the same effect you used to, you're treating the symptoms, not the cause...

Healing is automatic if you give your body a chance...

The food you ate in the past determines how healthy you will be in the future...

Too much protein is hazardous to your health...

You have the ability to improve your health... If you eat more protein daily than the equivalent of one hamburger and two eggs, you're headed for chronic disease...

Our country's health care system is programmed to treat disease, not to promote health...

Urine with an ammonia odor is a warning sign that you are sick...

Americans spend about $500 BILLION a year on health care—that's nearly $2000 for every person.

Before We Begin, How Healthy Are You?

To achieve a goal of good health, you must know how healthy you are when you start. You can do a simple test at home that will tell you where you are now so you can map your journey to health.

Every morning when you get up and stumble into the bathroom, your body is ready to dispose of material it can't use. The vehicle used to eliminate this material — urine — offers clues to how your body responded to the food you ate yesterday. It also provides your best clue yet as to how you can expect to feel in the future.

The test described in this book isn't a diagnostic aid to tell you what's wrong with you — that's the responsibility of your health care specialist. This book is your guide to find out how healthy you are!

All you need is some pH paper that registers above and below neutral — roughly between pH 5.5 and 8.0. Before you do any testing, though, you need to set the stage. Tonight, eat a hefty portion of steak, hamburger, chicken, grains, breads, pasta, or similar "industrial strength" food. Skip all vegetables and fruit. Load up on protein.

Tomorrow, right after you get up, catch some urine in a small, clean container and test it with a strip of the pH paper.

For most people, one of two things will happen to the paper. It will (1) change color dramatically, becoming very dark, or (2) the paper will appear only to be wet — not change color at all.

The color of the paper is your key to beginning to understand just how healthy you are. If your pH paper turned very dark,
1. you are not healthy even if you feel good, and
2. you must not engage in strenuous exercise.
If the pH paper didn't change color at all,
1. you are headed for serious disease if you continue this way;
2. you can still exercise.
You may see a definite change in the color of the paper, but it isn't to a deep, dark color. In that case, you can assume that right now you are still reasonably healthy and can continue to exercise.

Later in this book you will learn how to establish a more precise health index by a more detailed monitoring schedule. You'll also learn why you have reached your particular level of health, be it high or low.

With this quick, simple test, your body provides evidence of how well it is working. The following chapters will tell you how to interpret the evidence.

"Feeling good" and "being healthy" are not necessarily the same. However, you don't have to wait for symptoms of disease to tell you that something is wrong. Most of us wait until we're sick to worry about health. That's not the time to try to get healthy; that's the time to try to survive. You get healthy one day at a time.

You can improve your health; and by using a little strip of pH paper and a small sample of urine you'll know where you stand now and how far you have to go.

Prologue

Good health is available to everyone! Not just to the affluent. Not just to the well-educated. Not just to the well-insured. Everyone! Health is in the individual, not in pills, surgery, or "medicine."

In 1986, the people of the United States spent over $458 billion on health care. That is 10.9% of our gross national product, and averages out to approximately $1,837 for every man, woman, and child in the country. Cardiovascular disease alone accounted for over 88 billion health-care dollars in 1989. You would think that with that much money being dedicated to health we would be a nation of robust, energetic, vibrant individuals. But are we? Apparently not. Each year we spend more and more to try to fix body parts that have gone wrong.

We are a nation obsessed with illness. When two or more are gathered together in a social setting, the conversation turns into a friendly scrimmage of symptom one-upsmanship. Who had the highest fever during the last bout of flu? How strong was the medicine the doctor prescribed? Who was "down and out" the longest? What are the odds against full recovery, or the chances of long-term repercussions? From insomnia to arthritis or allergies to viruses, misery has become something of a status symbol. We seem to take perverse pleasure in seeing how un-well we can make ourselves without slipping over the edge to self-destruction. This is backwards! Where is it written that illness is mandatory? In contradiction to our attitude that illness is a normal part of life, a society exists where the people not only survive to be over one hundred years old, they live mentally and physically active lives well past the century mark.

The people of Hunza, hidden away in the Himalayas, are living testaments to the concept that health is a natural state of life. In this small, remote, independent state of Pakistan, there are no doctors, infant mortality is "virtually nonexistent," there are no childhood diseases or ulcers, and ninety-year-old men father children. For recreation, volleyball games pit the "youngsters" of 16 to 50 against the "elders" who are over 70 and as old as 145.

There are no crimes, jails, police, taxes, or banks, and essentially no divorces. The people live long, happy, satisfying, productive lives in harmony with themselves, each other, and their environment. They enjoy life and health.

What does this apparently idyllic society have to do with our fast-paced, ultra-modern, high-tech way of life? It illustrates that the human body will function well for decades longer than we give it credit for if we provide it the proper exercise, serenity, diet, and environment.

The primary personal responsibility of each of us is to promote our own health, not merely fight disease. We cannot do our best for ourselves, our families, communities, or society if we are constantly waging a no-win war against the symptoms of illness.

This book is about wellness and health — not disease crisis management. If you need pills or surgery to relieve painful symptoms, something is wrong with the way your body is functioning. Taking more pills won't correct the problem. Pills may mask symptoms and make you feel better, but pills and potions can't "cure." I believe that when you reach the point where you need drugs or surgery, you are in a crisis situation. Your body is not functioning as it was designed to function. You are not healthy!

To be sure, medicine has a vital job to do. It's important that we understand what this job is. Medicine's principal objective is to relieve pain and suffering — to make people more comfortable. Medicine provides the "fix-it" shop for the human body. Through drugs and surgery, the body's operating environment is altered. The purpose, if not the effect, of the alterations is to reduce discomfort or increase efficiency. But rarely, if ever, can chemical or surgical tinkering by even the most educated, intelligent, and skilled practitioner replicate the perfection of the original design.

Medicine can't heal. Drugs can't heal. Chiropractic can't heal. Only the body can heal. We can't do any more for the body than the body can do for itself. Over a decade ago, Dr. Beverly Winikoff of the Rockefeller Foundation in New York advised a Senate Select Committee on Nutrition and Human Needs of the fallacy of depending upon medicine to cure our individual or collective ills. The published report quotes Dr. Winikoff:

> *There is a widespread and unfounded confidence in the ability of medical science to cure or mitigate the effects of such [nutrition-related] diseases once they occur. Appropriate public education must emphasize the unfortunate but clear limitations of current medical practice in curing the common killing diseases. Once hypertension, diabetes, arteriosclerosis of heart disease are manifest, there is, in reality, very little that medical science can do to return a patient to normal physiological function.*

Your body will always do everything it can to continue to function. It recognizes the things that aren't right: areas that aren't demonstrating the perfection with which the body was created. Given the opportunity, the body will immediately start to repair injured or impaired areas. The critical stipulation is that it must be given the opportunity. Obviously, continuing activities, habits, and the lifestyle that brought about the distress isn't giving the body an opportunity to do anything differently.

If you break out in hives every time you eat strawberries and you hope for a different outcome as you continue to eat them, you can be almost certain nothing will change. You'll continue to break out. If your body is "malfunctioning," it is happening for a reason. You need to change the circumstances that brought about the malfunction before the body can heal itself. If you wear shoes that are two sizes too small, you will definitely get the impression that there is something wrong with your feet. You can take aspirin to relieve the pain, but that is hardly a solution to the problem. Pain is a protest by your body that it is being subjected to abuse. The problem that causes the pain stems from the conditions under which you are requiring your body to function.

I don't treat disease. I don't cure anybody of anything. The body does the curing. For example, a patient came to me after being told by a doctor that she had a serious blood disease and could expect to live only another three months. She decided to give her body a chance to respond to different foods and a different lifestyle than those she had previously inflicted on it. That was two years ago, and she still drops in to see me on occasion. Another patient came to me after he had been told by his doctor that he had about thirty days to live. That was nine years ago! I didn't cure him. He did what he needed to do to reverse the effects of the things he had been doing wrong. That's why he is still around.

I don't believe there is any disease you can't get over, as long as you understand the law of miracles. I once saw a sign that succinctly expresses my attitude: "I don't BELIEVE in miracles; I DEPEND on them."

I want to study how miracles work. I don't think they should happen only once in a while. They should happen constantly. Yet if man can't explain "spontaneous remissions," he chalks them up to a "misdiagnosis" or exaggerated claims.

The overall health of the people of this country is deplorable. The United States — the richest country in the world — is eighteenth in infant mortality. There are seventeen other countries in this world where your children or grandchildren have a better chance of surviving infancy. Figures from 1986-87 show that 10 out of every 1000 babies born in the United States die. Young adults in apparently top physical condition suddenly die. We are told that we are conquering cancer, yet children and young adults — 8-, 13-, and 26-year olds — are still dying of that disease.

Statistics can be found to support opposing claims that we are both winning and losing the war against cancer. In the January/February 1989 issue of *Hippocrates*, William Boly cites figures that refute the claim by the National Cancer Institute that cancer is being conquered. Despite this claim based on the percentage of patients "cured" of serious cancers, Boly reports "171 people per 100,000 succumbed in 1985, up from 162 in 1975 and 157 in 1950."

At what point are we going to say, "This isn't right!"? When are we going to stand up for our health rights and refuse to continue the expensive and often painful pattern of symptom chasing? Will it be when health care costs reach 50%, 75%, or 90% of the GNP?

Usually, we don't know what it is we did wrong that made us sick. The purpose of this book is to help you understand how food and lifestyle affect particular physiological functions that ultimately affect your health. It will give you a method to find out what your personal health index is right now. If you find you aren't really as healthy as you thought you were, it will help you understand why, and it will guide you on a course for correction. It will give you a clue as to what you have been doing that has prevented you from reaching your greatest health potential. On the other hand, if you are in fantastic health, it will help you to understand how your body works, what you can expect in the future, and how to continue on a life-long, health-improving, long-life track.

This book is not an instruction manual on how to chemically tinker with health by adding a little of this or a lot of that. It offers an explanation you haven't had before of why your body responds the way it does to some of the things you do to it. You will be introduced to a method of checking to see how your body has held up under the lifestyle it has had so far.

This book is not, nor is it intended to be, a "handy guide to a quick cure," or a "home remedy" manual. I am not offering a substitute for "medicine." I am offering information that can lead the reader to begin to rebuild his level of health as he continues to follow his doctor's directions for addressing health-crisis situations.

The descriptions of chemical reactions and processes presented in this book are, to the best of my knowledge, scientifically accurate. However, you won't find in other texts many of the concepts and conclusions concerning the body's response to these processes that are presented here. This explains precisely why most of us are in our current deplorable state of steadily declining health whether we feel good or not. We have been doing the best we can with the information we have had. Unfortunately, the "best" hasn't been nearly good enough to keep us free of unnecessary disease and pain.

By integrating my clinical experience and observations with my background in chemistry, physiology, and other "hard" sciences, I reached my conclusions of how following the high-protein myth is devastating human health. I have taken accepted scientific premises, held them up to the light of clinical results, and have gained a clearer picture of how diet affects your health. Nobel Prize winner Albert Szent-Gyorgyi is credited with saying: "Discovery consists of seeing what everybody has seen and thinking what nobody has thought."

My purpose is to offer an adjunct to current health care practices. No one should, on the basis of the information contained in these pages, discontinue any medications or treatments prescribed by a licensed health practitioner.

The medical community provides vital life-saving procedures for patients in acute distress. The concepts presented in the pages that follow are in no way intended to discount the importance and need for conventional medical treatment. Crisis intervention is often the only means of returning to a state where you can begin to take stock of your health situation and determine that something you were doing just wasn't giving you the outcome you wanted.

By understanding how the systems of the body work together, you will be in a better position to build a firm foundation of good health. The people of the tiny kingdom of Hunza have shown that we can live long, comfortable, energetic, productive lives. The attitude that aging is a "disease" is contrary to the design of life. Daily living need not be an exercise in progressive deterioration. No matter what your health status or age is right now, you can begin to take steps that will give your body that crucial "opportunity" to begin to repair itself.

We all know we have a finite life span. Yet we have accepted that everything "goes downhill after thirty." Your body is equipped to replenish and repair itself until it stops functioning altogether. You can give your body the golden opportunity to continue to get better whether you are currently in your "youthful" years, your "middle" years, or your "golden" years.

A fundamental premise of this book is that you have control over your health. I'm here to guide you on a trip to wellness. Only you can decide to make the journey.

CHAPTER 1

Introduction

You may be reading this introduction to decide whether or not to read the entire book. No matter what your decision, there is something you need to know. You are probably eating too much protein to be healthy! If your daily diet includes more protein than the equivalent of two eggs and a hamburger, your health is going downhill—fast! When protein makes up more than about twenty-five percent of your daily fare, you're getting too much. The rest of this book is to tell you why, and what you can do to reverse the damage that has already been done.

It is a book for anyone who has had enough of being sick or of not feeling as good as he would like. It's for all those who drag out of bed in the morning wondering why they are just as tired as they were the night before. And it's for those fortunate individuals who bounce out of bed every day feeling great.

It was written for you if you want to *be in control of your health!* In these pages, you will find principles of wellness no one else has told you. You will get a new perspective on how and why your body does the things it does. You will learn a simple, inexpensive, self-administered method of accurately measuring just how healthy you really are. It's time you were given a method of developing a complete picture of your health and clues as to why you may hurt or be tired all the time. After reading this book, you will be able to answer the perplexing question "why" that is raised when a friend or neighbor who felt great one day suffered an unexpected heart attack the next.

1

I'll explain how the great American tradition of a well-balanced diet, made up of the "basic four" food groups, has set you on a course to slow—often painful and certain—self-destruction.

Sound radical? It came as a surprise to me, too, when I realized where the research I was doing was leading. It led to concepts that take the mystique out of health. This is how it happened.

Over twenty years ago, I began devoting my energies to what I saw as "making sick people well." My health care practice had grown rapidly, and *most* of my patients improved greatly. Being a member of a profession that treats the body as a whole, I understood that when my patients improved, it was their own innate healing power that deserved the credit. I couldn't "heal" anyone! The body is a self-healing, self-regulating, unified creation that never makes a mistake. Every process, function and activity of the body is the perfect response for conditions the body faces at that moment.

There is a saying in the chiropractic profession: "The power that made the body can heal the body." The power that built the body from a single fertilized egg doesn't suddenly turn off at birth. Yet my clinical experience indicated that this innate power seemed to work on an erratic, part-time schedule. Some patients responded to treatment quickly and completely; others didn't respond nearly as well. That wasn't logical. I knew then as I know now, *everything the body does is completely logical.* There is not the slightest doubt about that! With this philosophy as a base, I began to investigate a major factor in everyone's life—food.

At that time, in the late '60s and early '70s, chiropractic colleges didn't pay much more attention to nutrition than medical schools did. But I had been well-schooled in "home style" and farm-family nutrition. My instincts and culture told me that patients who ate good, wholesome, well-balanced meals—whole wheat bread, whole milk, steak and potatoes—were the ones whose bodies allowed their innate self-healing qualities to put things right, after only one or two adjustments. It followed then that patients who ate primarily fast-food burgers, fries, and soft drinks were the ones who did not respond quickly.

To prove my theory, I began a study of my patients' food consumption habits. This study may go on record as having been one of the shortest nutrition investigations ever. After about three weeks, it became clear that the opposite of my expectations was being proved.

Much to my surprise, it was the folks who had coffee and donuts for breakfast, a sandwich and cola drink for lunch, and pizza or macaroni and cheese for dinner who got better faster.

This evidence really upset my cultural beliefs. As a dedicated health care practitioner, I faced a serious dilemma. I wasn't sure why pasta and pizza patients had a better track record for improvement than the conscientious "good food" eaters, but I certainly couldn't advise my steak and eggs patients to switch to donuts and peanut butter.

I didn't know as much about nutrition then as I do now; however, it was apparent that neither diet was "good." Patients who followed the traditional "well-balanced" diet were sicker than those who ate "junk food." The big question was, "Why?"

I began my odyssey into nutrition by canvassing the latest in nutrition information at the health food stores. What an assortment! You could find a book that would tell you just about anything you wanted to hear about which foods you should eat to be slim, smart, and happy—and to live to a ripe old age. Vegetables, fats, protein, grapefruit—you name it, and there was a book to give you a magic cure.

Obviously, I wasn't going to find what I needed there, so it was back to the text books from my undergraduate and graduate school days. Certainly, biochemistry, physiology, and anatomy would give me the answers I was looking for.

I read and compared various opinions of scholarly authorities, and related them to the things I had learned in my years in science, education, and clinical practice. The pieces of the puzzle began to come together.

The most startling conclusion was that *excess protein is the primary culprit in the health woes of Americans today.* Too much protein—that time-honored foundation of nutrition—puts such radical physiological stress on the body that the natural healing process is sabotaged. This, in turn, sets us up for developing the chronic diseases that plague our population.

When I speak of "excess protein," I'm not talking about the concentrated, high-protein concoctions that were credited with about sixty deaths in the '70s. I'm talking about the amount of protein you get from a daily diet of beef, pork, chicken, fish, eggs, beans, grains, nuts, pizza, spaghetti, bread, hamburgers, and the rest of our everyday foods. When these foods make up most of your diet, your body is put under intense nutritional stress. To process all of the protein, your body must adjust the way it works. After these adjustments have gone on for years, cells lose their ability to function the way they were intended, resistance is lowered, and disease is inevitable. Despite the body's ingenious self-regulating talents, any physiological system can be overloaded.

You are about to see—for the first time—*why* the food you eat makes you sick. Magazine and newspaper articles as well as radio and TV commentators tell about different substances that have been found to cause particular diseases in people or laboratory animals. Now, I am going to explain *why* disease comes about; how the food you eat day in and day out can contribute to your health problems; and what you can do to head disease off at the pass. All of these concepts are based on accepted scientific findings, blended with the certainty that the body never does anything wrong, and topped off with a refreshing dose of logic.

CHAPTER 2

The Good News and Bad News About Health

Did anyone ever come right out and tell you that you don't have to develop some sort of disease or live in pain? Well, I'm telling you now. The Good News is you don't have to be sick to be in style!

The Bad News is that just about everyone we know—family, friends, work-mates, your banker, plumber, and the neighbors down the street—all have problems with their health. You name it: allergies, bronchitis, cancer, depression, emphysema, fatigue... You can go right through the alphabet down to yaws and zygomycosis with names for different ways to be sick.

I'll say it again emphatically—*you don't have to be sick!*

Even though just about everyone seems to be sick or suffer in one way or another, you don't have to participate—unless you want to. You have a chance and a choice to be as healthy as you decide to be. Believe me, I'm not promising an overnight cure for anything. Without realizing it, you may have been laying the foundation for disease for years. However, *you really do have the ability to help yourself feel better and be healthy*—and you won't have to turn your whole life upside down to do it.

And more Good News. You can find out what your level of health really is and keep tabs on it, right in the privacy of your own home.

That's what this book is all about: Health, not disease. It's to show you:

- that you can take charge of your own health by learning how healthy you are right now;

- why you may be in less than glowing health; and

- how little effort it takes to improve and keep improving once you realize this first wellness principle:

WELLNESS PRINCIPLE: *Good health is natural!*

I am convinced that the body is infinitely intelligent. My nutrition research and twenty-five-plus years of clinical practice have shown me that our bodies are the smartest things around. Everything they do is not only logical but best for us at the time. *Your body doesn't know how to be sick; it knows exactly what to do to survive as long as possible.*

WELLNESS PRINCIPLE: *Your body isn't programmed to develop disease.*

Everything that happens in your body is caused by something. There is not one cell, not one bit of tissue, not one organ or system in your body that is designed to make you sick. Every function and process of your body is a response to a stimulus—the old "cause and effect" pattern. Furthermore, *every response of your body is perfect for the stimulus that caused it.*

Your body doesn't set goals to develop colitis, diabetes, or allergies. Your body responds in precise ways to every circumstance. If the response causes problems, we call the problems "symptoms." We give certain sets of symptoms labels signifying a particular "disease." Names like osteoporosis, AIDS, cancer, or arthritis are really just shorthand for a particular pattern of symptoms. Symptoms are the signals that the body is adapting its functions to survive the things we do to it. *Your body doesn't know how to be sick!*

Over the years, you have absorbed ideas about health and nutrition. You may have been led to believe that your body really doesn't know what it's doing. Most of us are conditioned to believe that we are at the mercy of luck and heredity to determine how healthy we are now and how sick we can expect to be in the future.

Up until now, you may have assumed that you have little control over your own health—that you are destined to get the same diseases as your forefathers. In reality, *you, and only you, are responsible for your own health.* Heredity plays an important role in how disease is manifested—cancer, diabetes, arthritis, and so forth—but heredity doesn't dictate that you *must* get sick. In other words, if you live in such a way that disease is inevitable, heredity will decide which form your particular disease will take.

We take for granted that for most occasions when our bodies act up, relief is as near as the closest pharmacy. And as far as "nutrition" is concerned, that's what you get from pizza made with whole wheat flour rather than white flour. Good nutrition may also mean restricting consumption of sweets, or adding a vegetable by putting lettuce on sandwiches. You may have stayed reasonably symptom-free despite these lax health-maintaining guidelines, but good health involves more than subduing the symptoms of heartburn or depending on luck and heredity; and there's more to nutrition than eating a BLT.

> **WELLNESS PRINCIPLE:** *The food that fuels your body this year dictates how healthy you will be in coming years.*

To get down to the basics of health, illness has only three causes. There are lots of variations in the way to be sick, but only three causes of any of them. I term these causes Toxicity, Timing and Thoughts. Everything that happens in the body can be traced to at least one of them.

Any one of the three can cause all sorts of symptoms, aches, and pains to appear. Often, though, at least two and probably all three are involved. I'll go into these in more detail later, but for now:

> **WELLNESS PRINCIPLE:** *"Health" is more than the absence of pain.*

I'm not saying that there is no such thing as disease or pain. I am a doctor and I see examples of these in my office every day. However, when you realize that all illness comes from the *responses* the body must make to stimuli—the type of food you eat, the kinds of stress you subject it to, and your attitudes—you will look at symptoms for what they are—*symptoms are warning signs that you have pushed your body's natural healing potential too far.*

You are the one to decide how you are going to live, what you are going to eat, and what you are going to think about. You have the choice of whether or not you are going to abuse your body. Only you can make your lifestyle decisions. You alone choose to over-exercise or under-exercise; eat too much or diet excessively; see how little sleep you can get by on for long periods; worry about things over which you have no control; drink too much; smoke; or do drugs.

Assuming you are in reasonable control of your day-to-day existence, no one else can force you to eat things that are not good for you, compel you to engage in activities that are harmful to you, or require you to dwell on the injustices, minor or major disasters, and personal slights that are part of everyday life. You are the decision maker for your life and health.

Anyone who is committed to taking responsibility for his own health can reach any level of wellness he wants. This is not to say that we can all develop physiques like Arnold Schwarzenegger, play tennis with the skill of Martina Navritolova, or pare down to ballerina size. There is a difference between physique and health. We can, however, improve our eating habits to reach our own highest levels of health.

WELLNESS PRINCIPLE: *You have control over your health.*

So there you have the basics of the Good News and the Bad News about health. When you get down to the rock-bottom, underlying causes of all diseases and illnesses, you find problems with Toxicity, Timing, or Thoughts. Your actions and reactions determine how healthy you are. When any of the three *T's* is out of sync, it can be put right. When you know what and where the problem is, you can do something about it.

This book focuses on Toxicity with only brief side-trips into Timing and Thoughts. We will talk about food and the acid levels of the body, how they are related, and the effects acid-producing foods have on the body in general and cells in particular.

Correcting the effects of years of dietary abuse, neglect and over-indulgence may be simple—but not easy. I can assure you that I know a whole lot more about nutrition than I find comfortable. If I hadn't become aware of what goes on in the body and how to correct it, I could have ambled merrily through life helping those I could and shrugging my shoulders helplessly over those I couldn't. Life would certainly have been less complicated that way—but not nearly as satisfying.

This is a self-health book to help you clean up your internal act so that your cells can work the way they were designed. We live and die at the cellular level. You can't be healthy if your cells are living in junk. And equally as important, I emphasize that you can be as healthy as you want. By using the simple self-test on page 92 of this book, you can tell how healthy you are now and how healthy you are likely to be in the future if you continue doing what you are doing.

Feeling good is a wonderful way to live. When you are healthy you not only feel good but you can enjoy life. You can be relaxed when you're watching TV or on vacation, be energetic in work or play, roll with personal or job-related "punches" more easily, and generally find that you wake up in the morning ready to go.

When you eat the foods your body can use best with the least amount of stress, you will find that good health is practically unavoidable. Your body really does know what it is doing!

CHAPTER 3

Germs and Colds

In the words of Gilbert and Sullivan, "Things are seldom what they seem."

Germs that we have been washing off, drowning in disinfectant, and tossing away with disposable tissues, are not the cause of disease. Furthermore, those recurring colds that send our comfort level down and our chicken soup consumption up are really signs that our bodies are taking care of themselves.

"Now hold on," I can hear you saying. "First you tell me protein is bad for me, then that my body doesn't know how to be sick; and now you're telling me that germs don't cause disease and that colds are good. Science has proved that colds and diseases like flu, mononucleosis, TB, and typhoid are triggered by germs of some sort. And I certainly don't feel like my body is doing me a favor when I have a cold."

Right, on all counts. But let's take a closer look at how germs affect health and what is going on when you have a cold. First, germs.

"Germs" are microorganisms, viruses, bacteria, and probably other life forms we don't even know about yet. Certainly, each can play a part in disease. But, they are not the *cause* of illness. When germs set up housekeeping in your body, they are merely exercising squatter's rights in warm, moist, comfortable quarters that feature an unlimited supply of food. Germs set up residence when your body's defenses are down.

WELLNESS PRINCIPLE: *Lowered resistance is the "welcome" sign for germs.*

Bacteria, viruses, and microorganisms are in and around us all the time. They don't show up just on rainy days, during winter, or when you get your feet wet. We live in a world teeming with microscopic activity. It's estimated that each of us carries about 10^{14} bacteria either internally or externally. That's 100 trillion of the little rascals. We are exposed to potential disease producers constantly; yet most of us are symptom-free much of our lives. With the concentration of germs in our immediate surroundings and in or on our persons, if they were the cause of disease, all of us would be sick incessantly. You have probably witnessed or experienced the "flu-bug" or colds running rampant through several members of a family while one or two stalwart souls escape the troublesome illness. If we were as susceptible to infection by germs as we have been led to believe, why is it that some members of the same household "catch" the current malady while others stay symptom-free? Are some of us just luckier than others? What about the survivors of the great plagues of history? Thousands of people died while many who cared for the sick and dying weren't infected. If each of us were to fall victim to every malevolent microorganism that came our way, none of us would have survived long enough to read (or write) these words.

When your body is really healthy—more than just symptom-free —disease-producing bacteria can't penetrate your defenses. All of the bacteria in your body aren't bad by a long shot. Some produce enzymes that break down food molecules into forms you can assimilate. Other bacteria produce pigment, and still others are active in essential chemical processes.

There are literally tons of bacteria in the soil. Although some soil bacteria get their nourishment from inorganic materials, most live on living or nonliving organic material. They contribute to ecology: they break down organic matter, participate in the nitrogen cycle, and enrich the soil. Many bacteria are beneficial to man and his environment.

Pathogenic bacteria, such as tetanus and botulinus, are subsets of bacteria that can produce disease in their host. From man's perspective, detecting a redeeming feature in these organisms is difficult.

Fortunately, science has come up with crisis intervention treatment for emergencies if we step on a rusty nail or eat improperly preserved foods when our resistance is low. Our best bet is to avoid being exposed to such mischief makers and to make sure we eat correctly so that our vitality and resistance are high enough to repel their effects if we inadvertently tangle with them.

Germs don't affect health unless they are able to penetrate the cells of an organism—really get into the working parts. Germs can't penetrate cells until the body's vitality and resistance are reduced. Then the cells are susceptible to invaders. An accident, the wrong kind of food, excessive fatigue, or high-intensity stress are all resistance reducers. Short-term, high-intensity events of an accident, or long-term, non-stop abuse of a destructive lifestyle disrupt the normal function of the body as a whole, as well as the cells that make up that whole.

The strategy for avoiding infectious disease is not to kill off all bacteria to avoid illness. The best course is to make sure your cells are healthy enough to keep your vitality at its peak. How vital are your cells? How "alive" are you? Your health, vitality, and resistance to disease is determined by the health of your cells.

WELLNESS PRINCIPLE: *Germs can't insist if the cells can resist.*

What, then, determines the health of your cells?

Lifestyle is the primary determinant of your health: what you eat, how rough you are on your body, how you rest, and what sort of attitude you have. Those whose diets consist of a lot of protein and few vegetables put their cells in a position of having to struggle for survival. If they are also hyperactive, grouchy worriers, they are prime candidates for chronic disease or early death.

A physiological response occurs every time any of your five senses is stimulated by food, activities, impressions, environment, attitudes, memories, arguments, anger, frustrations . . . And your cells are affected by every physiological response. Responses generated by positive stimuli such as good food, rest, and positive attitudes, are beneficial to your cells. Responses to negative stimuli such as physical and emotional trauma, negative attitudes, and toxin-producing foods sap the energy and vitality of your cells. When the vitality of your cells is reduced, the vitality of your whole body suffers and your resistance to disease is decreased. We live or die at the cellular level.

The fast-paced, high-stress lifestyles of many Americans are chock-full of stimuli that have harmful effects on cells. Cells that are not completely healthy aren't able to ward off attack—resistance goes down. When resistance is down, germs do a number on health.

Symptoms of pain, discomfort, fever, nausea, or other signs of disease develop according to the type of trauma inflicted on the body. Some symptoms, such as cuts and broken bones, are apparent immediately; others, like allergies and osteoporosis, take longer to show up. When symptoms are particularly uncomfortable (or when they interfere with the routine of daily living), the sufferer will usually look to a doctor for relief. If the person consults a medical doctor, drugs may be prescribed to combat the symptoms. Yet despite the fact that there is neither intelligence nor vitality in drugs, drugs bring about responses that may relieve symptoms. However, the problem that caused the symptoms is still there.

If bacteria are the cause of discomfort, antibiotics will often rout the offenders. Unfortunately, germs can adapt to their environment also, and more and more bacteria are becoming resistant to drugs that have previously kept them in line. Drugs may kill bacteria, but unless the resistance of the host is improved, the same or another variety of bacteria will strike again and gain another foothold. Most antibiotics are the essence of democracy—they go after helpful bacteria equally as vigorously as they go after harmful bacteria.

WELLNESS PRINCIPLE: *You can never treat enough symptoms to correct the cause.*

A living organism (such as your body) is greater than the sum of its parts. Every system of the body is made up of individual cells. Any time a cell does not perform to the benefit of the greater whole, the vitality of the system decreases. If a system can't function up to par, the body suffers. When the vitality, or vital force, of the body drops, resistance drops. The body as a whole is then susceptible to invasion and domination by germs.

When the germs find a congenial host, they begin to multiply. In cases such as malaria, the by-product of multiplication becomes so toxic that life is threatened.

Germs don't have the ability to dictate their actions or create their environment. They can survive only in an environment that is hospitable to them. Germs, like people, are survival oriented. They will find homes that offer the best opportunity for sustained existence and propagation.

Bacteria neither create nor control their environment or destiny. Bacteria multiply and grow in the environment in which they find themselves. In the body, the environment is determined by the host's lifestyle. If bacteria that belong in your garden take up residence in your lungs, you may perceive the intruders as "bad"—creatures of malice that must be destroyed. Actually, they are not "bad"; they are merely in the wrong place for our needs. They need to be relocated. There's no such thing as a "bad" germ. However, they, like people, can be in the wrong place at the wrong time. Those who have been an innocent party to a bank robbery know well what it means to be in the wrong place at the wrong time.

All pathogenic germs (those that are harmful to the body) are scavengers. They don't attack normal, vital, healthy cells or tissue. They can't feed on healthy cells. They can grow and prosper only when damaged cells serve as a generous host that provides ample nutrition and an accommodating environment.

Germs, including the alleged "cold germs," don't suddenly appear in our lives to cause us grief. They are around us and in us all the time. By keeping your body as fit as possible through diet, you will be able to peacefully co-exist with germs. They have as much right on this planet as we do.

Germs that invade the inner workings and hidden mechanisms of the body force the body to respond. The responses aren't pleasant—they are signs that the defenses are down.

WELLNESS PRINCIPLE: *Germs aren't the cause of disease—low resistance is.*

A runny-nose, watery-eye, miserable cold is an internal cleansing process. Your body will do everything it can to maintain its steady state of homeostasis. Its first line of defense against unwanted or unnecessary visitors is dilution. Diluting substances the body doesn't need renders them less harmful. The body will either dilute or try to evict harmful or unnecessary substances. One method of removing unwanted or toxic materials from the body is the common cold. A cold may make you feel rotten, but the cold itself serves a purpose. Your body is getting rid of toxins that can threaten your survival. As long as you can develop a good cold, your body is still able to fight. I've never known of a person in the final stages of cancer to have either a cold or a fever.

The fever that sometimes accompanies a cold and other ailments is another ingenious method of cleaning out the body. Fevers kill off intruders. Pathogenic bacteria fare best in a temperature of about 98.6° Fahrenheit. Consequently, a controlled fever (up to 104° F) can dispatch germs, burn off toxic material, and allow the body to resume its regular routine. Both science and culture acknowledge that fevers serve a health-restoring purpose; however, the pesky cold hasn't yet been awarded this status.

It isn't at all uncommon for colds to be more prevalent when fresh fruits and vegetables become more available and affordable in the late spring or summer. Eat a batch of watermelon or other fresh fruit and, unless you are walk-on-water healthy to begin with, you can be almost assured of coming down with that most bothersome of minor maladies—a "summer cold."

Nevertheless, colds serve much the same purpose as fevers: they clean out unwanted toxins. Diet may be the instigator of a constant succession of colds. High protein intake continually dumps toxins into your system, and your body will tolerate only so much accumulated toxin before its saturation point is reached. A good cold is one way to clean out some of the mess.

Cold symptoms can also be brought about by improving your diet too quickly and giving your body more naturally beneficial food than it is accustomed to handling. When this happens, your body isn't rebelling against excess toxicity. Instead, your cells are clearing out the remnants of excess protein faster than your elimination system can take the debris out of the body.

WELLNESS PRINCIPLE: *Colds are survival tactics.*

No matter how much money is spent trying to eradicate the common cold and nullify all of the microorganisms that are potential health threats, we'll never succeed. Since germs aren't the problem, killing them off isn't the solution. Every time you get a cold, as difficult as it may be through your runny nose and tears, you should be thankful that your body still has enough vitality to defend itself.

CHAPTER 4

The Intelligence Within

Remember when you were nothing more than a fertilized egg looking for a place to attach yourself? Of course you don't. There is no conscious direction involved in the development of an embryo. Neither you nor your mother had any conscious control over when it was time to install blood vessels, select eye and hair color, or generate fingernails for you.

So if neither you nor your mother devised a production schedule or supervised the project, who was in charge?

You had to develop either by plan or by randomness; there are no other choices. If each of us were a random proliferation of cells, even members of the same family would bear no resemblance to one another. We would see more variations among populations than just color of eyes, hair, and skin, or differences in size and shape. If there were no consistency in human development, some of us might have eyes on our shoulders, others a nose on each of five kneecaps, and some with an ear on one of the three fingers that bent backwards. No, you didn't develop by random proliferation of cells; you developed very systematically according to an established plan. An intelligence infinitely greater than the conscious mind of man has been in charge since before you were born—and, I might add, has done a masterful job.

My purpose is not to go into who or what devised and implemented the plan for developing the human body; it is to

17

acknowledge that we develop in a very specific manner. The same plan of embryonic development guided each of us. There is an innate intelligence in every person that keeps physiological processes on schedule from the very beginning.

Each of us has an internal intelligence that coordinates and synchronizes all of the functions of the wonderfully and incomprehensibly complex human body. The abilities of this intelligence dwarf the capabilities of the most sophisticated supercomputers. The systems-coordinating skills of electronic "super brains" that can dispatch and return space probes or send the stock market into an economy-rocking tailspin are cumbersome and primitive compared with the natural orchestrating talents of our built-in body wisdom. Under the direction of this sophisticated intelligence, the billions of bits and parts that constitute a unique individual can hum along for decades in fine-tuned harmony.

The same infallible director that brought each of us into existence from the union of sperm and egg oversees postnatal physical growth and repair. Throughout your life, cuts heal, broken bones knit, and hair and fingernails grow. The body's internal intelligence orchestrates these and thousands of other repair and replenishment activities without your giving them a single thought. Ordinarily, we aren't at all conscious of the continuous intricate physiological symphony that plays within our bodies from conception to death. However, when something is wrong, we become acutely aware of the discord.

WELLNESS PRINCIPLE: *The intelligence that made your body runs your body.*

The closest modern science has come to locating a physical area of this innate intelligence is in the DNA molecule. DNA carries the code for genetic information. However, everything we know about DNA still doesn't completely explain our development. For starters, how can one cell containing DNA multiply and keep multiplying only to have some of the new cells become skin, some bone, some nerve, and some muscle? The cells of all of these tissues are different and perform specialized functions, yet they all descended from the same original cell.

What prompts the cells to modify to become such an intricate network of a variety of tissue, organs, and systems? And how in the world does this happen *perfectly* the same way every time? Let's go back to the very beginning of each individual.

In the split second of fertilization, there is perfection! Instantly, perfection is expressed. From that split second of perfection comes a perfect human being, unless something interferes. Development may be less than perfect when the environment is not conducive to supporting the perfection that was created. Although perfection is flawless, it is not indestructible. It can be overridden when the contrivances of man's educated mind (including conscious selection of inappropriate food) interfere. Nevertheless, we were all perfect when we started out! At conception, we all had our split second of perfection.

As an extreme example of how environment can violate perfection, recall the tragedy of the thalidomide babies in the early '60s. Doctors prescribed pills to relieve the mothers' morning sickness. Although the morning sickness was a symptom of problems resulting from the mothers' life styles, the pills were to help them feel better— to relieve the symptoms. After taking the pills, the mothers did, indeed, feel better. But the chemicals in the pills interfered with the *natural* development of their babies. As a result, the expression of perfection at birth was less than the perfection at conception.

Products of the conscious mind of man can make absolutely no positive contribution to the development of an embryo into a normal, healthy baby! In fact, any conscious interference as a new life develops assures a problem.

WELLNESS PRINCIPLE: *The conscious mind of man is no match for the Intelligence Within.*

The same perfect intelligence that was present at conception guides the body's functions throughout life. It doesn't desert us or float off into the ionosphere when we are born. It keeps functioning instant by instant to keep us alive. Our internal intelligence keeps us going despite all of the abuse we heap on ourselves.

Before we were born, we were in a reasonably well-controlled environment. After we emerged into the world, we were faced with all manner of hazards: physical trauma, drastic temperature changes, good food, inappropriate food, no food, or too much food. The internal intelligence adapts the body's functions to accommodate to these and thousands of other variations just to keep us alive; and we aren't even conscious of it.

The wonderful thing is that accommodate it does! For every stimulus your body receives, whether it comes from inside or outside, the response is unfailingly perfect. When you're cold, the blood-flow to the skin is restricted in order to preserve body heat, and involuntary physical activity is initiated to generate heat—you shiver. When you're too warm, your body revs up its climate control system; it sends more blood to the skin area for cooling and pumps moisture through the skin for evaporation—you perspire. When you need more fuel to generate energy, messages are sent to your brain that you interpret as "hunger." When you eat something the body can't use, it gets rid of it. When . . . You get the idea. Everything that goes on in your body is a perfect response to a particular stimulus, and you never give it a thought until it happens. Now, that's Intelligence.

Just as our physical design was not haphazard or accidental, neither are our responses haphazard.

WELLNESS PRINCIPLE: *Every action and reaction in your body is perfect for the prevailing conditions.*

We are stimulus-response mechanisms. Everything that goes on in your physical being is in response to at least one stimulus.

I didn't originate this concept. We are told on TV talk shows and ads, in magazines, in newspapers, by "authorities" and friends about the responses we will get if we don't mend our ways. Eat high-cholesterol food and you'll develop heart problems; be a "couch potato" and your arteries will harden; smoke and you'll get lung cancer. We are also told, indirectly, that we can reorganize our not-too-smart bodies by manipulating their stimulus-response mechanisms with pills or potions: use Brand X to relieve constipation, Brand Y to relieve diarrhea, and Brand Z to take care of the hemorrhoids brought on by the other two. Brands X, Y, and Z are stimuli that cause the body to generate particular responses. Of course, the cause of the original problem hasn't been changed. The response that showed up as symptoms of the original problem has just been over-powered by the response to a more urgent stimulus. For a given stimulus, you get a given response—cause and effect.

As we will see later, you may not be aware of the stimulus that is causing a particular response that has been labeled with a name depicting a specific condition—osteoporosis, hives, parkinsonism— but the stimulus is there and the response to it is perfect. *The body never makes a mistake!*

WELLNESS PRINCIPLE: *Everything the body does is perfect for the conditions imposed on it.*

You may not like a physiological response if it makes you hurt or sick; nonetheless, the response is in your best interest—it is Natural, Normal, or Necessary.

Natural responses generally don't give you much trouble. You respond naturally (according to nature) to most daily situations. Your muscles contract or relax on cue, your pupils dilate and con-tract according to light intensity, food is processed uneventfully, your heart keeps a steady rhythm, cells die and are replaced—all of that sort of thing. When your lifestyle conforms to the natural scheme of things, your body isn't required to make an unusual num-ber of major adjustments. Unfortunately, most of us have adopted nutrition lifestyles that don't allow for exclusively natural physiologi-cal responses. However, since most of us in the U.S. eat essentially the same types of food (supermarket fare rather than wild boar, bam-boo shoots and berries) and follow relatively similar lifestyle patterns (climate controlled housing, automated transportation, and "high tech" living as opposed to cave dwelling), our bodies are adapting in similar ways.

When enough people are doing the same thing and it's no longer unusual, whatever they are doing becomes "normal." It's normal for us to have at least one TV in our home; it's normal for children to be inoculated; it's normal for people to develop osteoporosis as they get older; it's normal for urine pH to be between 4.5 and 8.0. As more and more people are found to exhibit a certain trait, that trait is labeled "normal," although it may not be natural. Generally, we use the term *normal* when we really mean *average* or *customary*. "Normals" that occur customarily are not necessarily the same as "normals" that occur naturally. Body temperature of 98.6 is a natural normal; tubes in babies' ears are becoming a *customary* normal.

The physiological responses that result in what we call disease, are neither natural nor normal—they are *necessary*. They happen because the body will always do whatever is necessary to survive. It must respond. Most of this book is devoted to showing how continuous necessary adaptations to excess protein in your diet can ensure disease. Long-term physiological adaptations that are absolutely necessary for immediate survival virtually guarantee disease.

Necessary functions of the body are adaptations the body *must* make to its natural way of doing things. Often the adaptations are quite natural along with being necessary. You are a pretty resilient specimen: you can adapt for short periods without grave consequences. For example, if you run full-tilt for a block to catch a bus, an increase in blood pressure and respiration is necessary to supply extra energy to your muscles and to get rid of the additional acid the exercise produces. But you have a problem if blood pressure and respiration don't return to normal soon after you sit down. If the necessary adaptations continue when you don't need them, you're headed for trouble.

Necessary adaptations are the work of your internal intelligence. They are ingenious safety devices. But when necessary adjustments become the norm, your body is not functioning naturally, and ultimately major problems will occur. The most major of these problems is premature death.

WELLNESS PRINCIPLE: *Every response of the body is normal, natural, or necessary.*

About now, a logical question for you to be asking is, "What does all of this internal intelligence, stimulus and response, survival, cells and conception have to do with the food we eat?" These concepts are all very important for understanding how your diet can require your body to adapt the way it normally functions. You will soon see that your intelligence within can handle just about anything you throw at it in the way of food. No matter what, it will keep you going as long as possible; *however,* you may not be happy with the by-products of the way it must work, and "as long as possible" may not be as long as you had planned.

We must keep in mind that the purpose of eating is to provide the body with the fuel needed to operate at its best for the longest period of time. Since we don't feed just our taste buds and appetites, it's helpful to have an overall picture of how the whole body works in order to understand why it responds the way it does to the way it is treated. One of the main points of this book is to help you to realize that your body never makes a mistake. Even if you are experiencing very unpleasant symptoms right this minute, the responses that caused the symptoms are perfect for the environmental conditions within your body.

This is probably an entirely different view of your health problems than you have had before. We have been conditioned to accept physical distress as a normal part of life. Actually, if your body operated the way it was designed, you couldn't fight off good health with a stick. Your intelligence within is that powerful.

CHAPTER 5

The Three Causes of Disease

Earlier, I introduced you to Toxicity, Timing, and Thoughts—the three causes of any disease no matter what label you put on it. I also stated that you have control over each of the causes.

It's entirely possible that you may view this concept with a bit of well-entrenched skepticism. Your reaction might be, "This fellow is really out in left field. I can name a bunch of causes of disease: bacteria, viruses, genetics, high cholesterol, high blood pressure, carcinogens, and just plain old age." And you would be absolutely correct—to a point. These *apparent* causes, plus many more, are merely character actors in the disease scenario. They are not the stars. They are among the "bad guys" that *appear* to be the culprits. However, they are not the back-to-square-one *causes* of disease. The stage has to be set for any of these dissidents to begin to make their effects known. They are the "terrorists" of the body that strike when there is no resistance. They may be present in a well-tuned, healthy body, but they are powerless against the impenetrable security system of the internal intelligence that maintains our resistance.

If disease were a "natural" consequence of life, we would all experience essentially the same ailments at about the same times of life. After all, we all follow roughly the same pattern of progress in our development: we teethe, learn to walk and talk, turn into a "terrible two," and suffer through the anguish of puberty at approximately the same ages. Although there are minor variations in the timing of the

24

onset for each of us, the pattern is pretty consistent. The development of disease, however, isn't consistent. Heart disease, arthritis, or
cancer, for example, can strike at any age.

Even the ravages of "old age" are inconsistent. The process of
aging isn't as neat and tidy as the process of developing from infant
to adult. There appears to be no particular "natural progression"
from young adulthood to old age. I have patients in their forties
who are "old." They think, feel, and act "old." And I have patients
in their nineties who have more vigor and vitality than others in
their fifties.

WELLNESS PRINCIPLE: *Age is no excuse for disease.*

Aging and disease are individual processes that are affected by
lifestyle. Your external, visible lifestyle is controlled by choices made
within personal boundaries of values, geography, and economics.
Your internal health-determining lifestyle is controlled by your personal Toxicity, Timing, and Thoughts.

This book is about Toxicity and how the food you eat contributes
to the build-up of toxins in your body. Toxins are poison-like substances. They can come from the air we breathe, liquids we drink,
things we eat, or substances we inject into our bodies.

Anything that goes into your body must be dealt with in some
way. Your body must use it, store it, or lose it. No "foreign" substance
in your body can be ignored, and until food is processed and assimilated, it is a "foreign" substance.

Essentially, this book gives you a new perspective on how your
body must adapt to take care of the elements in food that cause toxicity. Many food elements, such as vitamins, minerals, and enzymes,
are essential to health. However, excesses of even some of these beneficial elements can cause toxicity.

When I talk about "toxicity," I'm talking about the condition of
your cells. The cells in your body—liver cells, pancreas cells, heart
cells, and all of the rest—use glucose for energy; yet each type of cell
has a specific function to perform. The function of the heart cell is
contraction; the function of a parietal cell in the stomach is secretion
of hydrochloric acid. Every type of cell has a different function, but
each uses the same fuel—glucose—for energy. If the cells become

toxic and are not capable of functioning and utilizing that energy, disease begins.

Cells become toxic when they and their environment become too acid. Most of the fluids in your body where your cells are operating are supposed to be slightly alkaline.

WELLNESS PRINCIPLE: *We live or die at the cellular level.*

Your body is alkaline by design and acid by function. Although your cells live in an alkaline environment, they produce acid as they function.

Acid must be either neutralized or eliminated. Acid produced by cells is "natural," and self-made acid is easily eliminated through the lungs, the urine, and feces. Acid from foods is handled quite differently. There are intricate systems to neutralize dietary acid (more about acid, alkaline, and neutralization later). The body can handle reasonable quantities of dietary acid. However, too much acid-producing food overloads neutralizing mechanisms; the environment of your cells deteriorates; and your body becomes overly acid—it becomes toxic. Too much acid is termed acidosis. ACIDOSIS = TOXICITY.

Any substance that interferes with the *natural* workings of the body is a toxin—food included!

As we have seen, toxins are sometimes eliminated by natural, periodic cleansing procedures we call colds and fevers. You don't "catch" a cold or "come down" with a fever; you *earn* them. The body is getting rid of toxins. When you realize that colds are beneficial physiological processes, you can then understand why science has been unable to find the long sought-after cure despite the megabucks poured into research.

If you can't get rid of toxins from foods through natural processes, your body adapts the function of some of the cells. Sustained necessary adaptations reduce a person's resistance and set the stage for disease.

In our society, one of the principle sources of physiological toxins is *too much protein*. Excess protein doesn't have the immediate poisonous effect of strychnine or cocaine. However, when you eat more protein than your body needs to function optimally, a series of physiological changes is initiated. As we shall see in the following chapters, it's those changes that can lead to all manner of complaints.

WELLNESS PRINCIPLE: *Too much protein leads to toxicity.*

The second villain that undermines health and is a major cause of pain is improper internal Timing.

Your body synchronizes an amazing number of functions. It simultaneously keeps the blood coursing through your veins, digests foods, assimilates nutrients, eliminates unusable parts of foods, contracts and relaxes muscles, processes chemicals, repairs itself—the list goes on. You stay relatively symptom-free as long as all of the natural physiological functions work smoothly. That's Intelligence.

Sometimes, however, the timing of one of these functions isn't appropriate for the conditions of the moment. The concept of inappropriate timing can be explained by an illustration from daily life. Brushing your teeth is a "correct" action. It helps to preserve your teeth, keep your mouth clean, and avoid the pain that comes with dental neglect. However, brushing your teeth during a job interview isn't appropriate. There's nothing wrong with the activity itself—but the timing can be inappropriate.

To convert that analogy to your physiology, when you run or exercise hard, your heart rate increases. This is a natural, normal, and necessary function to increase the oxygen supply to your muscles and to remove the waste products from them. If your heart weren't able to increase its rate when needed, you wouldn't have survived your first chase around the playground. However, for your heart to continue to beat at the faster rate after you have rested is inappropriate; if it does, your body is experiencing a timing problem.

Most of my patients come to me for relief of symptoms brought about by incorrect timing. Muscles that should be relaxed are tense. Of course, if we couldn't tense our muscles, we wouldn't be able to move. However, when a patient is lying on an examination table, he should be able to consciously relax his voluntary muscles. A muscle that is continuously tense eventually becomes painful. Pain can be brought on by a perfectly proper physiological response that occurs at an inappropriate time.

You may wonder why the body would do something at the wrong time if its internal intelligence never makes a mistake. Doing the right thing is never a mistake—inappropriate maybe, but not wrong. The body doesn't judge an event good, bad, or appropriate. It just responds normally to all stimuli without judging whether or not the time is appropriate to execute the response. The information available to your control center serves as the data base for patterns of response to every situation. The brain that directs everything that goes on in the body works with the information recorded there. Information recorded yesterday, last month, twenty-, thirty-, or sixty-years ago is equally as usable as information recorded now, twenty-, thirty-, or sixty-seconds ago.

The response pattern is similar to retrieving data stored on a personal computer's hard disk. The computer doesn't care when the information was entered. It's either there or it's not there. When the computer gets a particular sequence of commands (the stimulus), it will retrieve the data associated with those commands (response). The body (like the PC) doesn't evaluate the appropriateness or potential long-term consequences of responses to stimuli. The body (like the computer that doesn't give a rip about health) does not consider health or disease. The body responds to stimuli from a data base (memory bank) that is programmed for survival at the moment. Pain and health problems arise when your body responds to stimuli from past conditions that no longer exist—obsolete programming.

I've seen thousands of examples of this over the years. A patient (we'll call him Jim) comes to me complaining of back or neck pain. He had been in a minor accident several weeks earlier. He may have been in a car that was rear-ended with only enough force to damage the bumper. Or he could have merely moved a dining room table. Or perhaps he just bent over to pick up the morning paper and he couldn't straighten up again. Whatever the incident that caused the pain, it wasn't an earth shaking event. But here he is, weeks later, still hurting.

A thorough examination shows nothing torn, nothing broken, nothing dislocated—just activity-restricting, sleep-disturbing pain.

It doesn't take long to recognize that Jim's body is still physiologically primed to handle the bumper-thumper, or lifting the table, or bending over. When he is lying on the treatment table "consciously relaxed," his muscles are more tense than they should be. Although the need for a physiological "alert" pattern is long gone, Jim's body is responding to the obsolete messages.

All that is necessary for Jim's muscles to relax is to update the messages his subconscious mind is sending his muscles. With updated signals, his muscles can relax. When this is done, pain is relieved. Jim can go on about his business, and his body can return to its non-emergency mode of function instead of the crisis/survival mode it had been maintaining.

WELLNESS PRINCIPLE: *The body works only for immediate survival, not toward long-term health and happiness.*

We have a survival instinct that has served mankind well. In order to withstand threatened attacks, the body goes into what we call *defense physiology*.

You may not be consciously aware that your body is responding to events of the past, but these buried memories may keep your body in defense physiology without you knowing it. In time, you will begin to experience pain and develop symptoms of illness, all because your memory patterns are keeping your body in an up-tight survival mode rather than allowing it to respond to the stimuli of the moment. Your body is in a defensive state and accumulating more acid than it can handle effectively. Thoughts exert the most powerful influence on your health, and *negative thoughts are the #1 acid producer in your body*.

WELLNESS PRINCIPLE: *Emotional stress in the form of negative thoughts can have painful consequences.*

The impact of thoughts on the musculoskeletal system was painfully illustrated recently when a patient came to my clinic for relief from back pain that had started the day before. In the course of our conversation he said, "I don't know if this has anything to do with it, but my wife lost her job ten days ago, and today is her last day. Two days ago my boss told me I'm losing mine in two weeks."

It's not hard to imagine how this fellow's thoughts were affected. He knew that it took two incomes to satisfy his family's standard of living, and in two weeks there would be no income. He hadn't really done anything unusual physically that would have caused back pain, but his thoughts had put his physiology in a defense mode. His body was on guard, ready to defend his family and himself. He knew they were in danger, but the enemy was invisible.

He was in a stressful situation. His body was responding in precisely the correct manner; however, the emergency showed no signs of letting up. Even though neither he nor his family was without food or shelter at the time, he was anticipating *with strong feelings of emotion* all sorts of dire consequences: defaulted mortgage, cars repossessed, major reductions in the trappings of affluence, personal embarrassment, and worse. And his body was ready for the physical fight that would never come.

Your body reacts to negative mental and emotional stress brought about by thoughts exactly the same way it reacts to "real" threats of physical harm. To the subconscious that governs physiology, stimuli from ideas are just as "real" as stimuli generated by being the target of a marauding street gang. Thoughts are things that can stimulate physiological responses—some appropriate for the occasion, some inappropriate. Physiologists have found that thoughts are so influential that all you have to do is anticipate exercise for the sympathetic nervous system to stimulate cardiac output.[1]

Timing, toxicity, and thoughts are closely interwoven. Rarely do I see a patient who doesn't have a problem with at least two of these factors, and most come to me with a combination of all three. Over time, any one of the three can force the body to adapt the way it functions, which in turn, leads to exhaustion, lowered resistance, and, ultimately, disease.

CHAPTER 6

Eating Your Way to Better Health

Stress-producing Thoughts are the most potent toxin producers in your body. Foods are in second place. This book is about how the food you eat can increase toxicity in your body and how to convert your degenerating eating patterns into a regenerating lifestyle.

We usually eat foods we enjoy. We generally enjoy foods that have the tastes and consistencies familiar to us. For the most part, we like what we are used to—corned beef and cabbage, Yorkshire pudding, raw fish, pasta, warm beer. Geography plays a large part in the formation of our food preferences. For the most part, our tastes cater to food "like mother used to make." Occasionally we enjoy (or profess to enjoy) cross-culture foods that are in vogue. However, essentially our tastes are pretty much defined by our individual backgrounds. We Americans may live on hamburgers and pizza much of the time, but at holidays, such as Thanksgiving or the Fourth of July, we celebrate by "pigging out" on the traditional foods of turkey, hot dogs, or other childhood favorites.

WELLNESS PRINCIPLE: *Tastes are developed, not inherited.*

Yet most of us have, at one time or another, determined to "improve" our eating habits. Before undertaking a diet change, you need to ask yourself, "Why am I doing this?" Your motivation for altering

31

what you eat, or any other important aspect of your lifestyle, is one of the most crucial factors in reaching whatever goal you have set.

Rarely do we do anything that doesn't have some sort of personal payoff. Each of us has his own reason for consciously deciding to alter a major facet of lifestyle. Some lifestyle changes are directed toward a specific goal: losing weight to look and feel better; stopping smoking to reduce health risks; or changing jobs to progress financially and professionally. Some changes are prompted by more nebulous motivators: a search for "something better"; happiness; or personal satisfaction.

Most people who are afflicted with life-threatening illness are eager to undertake any change that offers a glimmer of hope of improving their circumstances. Those who suffer pain or chronic discomforts are generally motivated to try just about anything to relieve their symptoms. Health-conscious individuals are ever on the alert for new and better ways to improve the quality and length of their lives. And millions of people are constantly looking for a simple way to lose weight. The reason you change your diet and the degree of your devotion to reaching your goal are paramount to your success.

Often, when we embark on a new diet plan or health regimen, our good intentions falter under pressure from our taste buds. We tend to eat the foods we want rather than those some "authority" tells us are "good for us."

Although we have a tendency to lapse into our dietary comfort zone despite our noble intentions, the transition to a more advantageous way of eating for a lifetime of health doesn't need to be overwhelming or traumatic. You are the one who decides what you are going to eat. A commitment to health is a personal pledge; all I can do is to give you the information that will help you fulfill your commitment. It's up to you to treat your body in a way that it can best take care of itself. By understanding the "ideal" nutrition plan, you'll have a goal to shoot for. Dissatisfaction with your present state of health can spur you to begin to improve your diet. Evidence that your efforts are being rewarded can keep you on track.

You don't have to become a vegetarian to be healthy. Your body can handle moderate amounts of most foods. It can also *occasionally* handle overly-generous quantities of foods that can cause problems. High-protein foods—meats, dairy products, and grains—that are the foundation of most Americans' diets are the champion toxin producers. If you limit heavy protein consumption to special occasions, such as holidays, your metabolic processes can roll with the punches.

WELLNESS PRINCIPLE: *Eating feeds more than our bodies.*

Eating is an integral part of our culture. We use eating to satisfy physical, emotional, and social hungers. We eat with other people both to please our palates and to enhance social or business relationships. Rare indeed is the social gathering that doesn't provide food of some sort. From serve-yourself chips and dip or cheese and crackers to tuxedo-clad-waiter-served full-course formal meals, we signal our camaraderie by serving or accepting food. There's no doubt about it—food is a major force in our lives.

Since we are all going to eat, we may as well include in our normal diets those things that will do the most to keep us healthy, and save the "treats" for special occasions.

Your goal for healthful eating is to arrange your daily fare so that about 75% of it provides the nutrients necessary to handle the other 25%. That boils down to daily menus of about 75% fruits and vegetables and about 25% high-protein meat, dairy, and grain products. As a people, our diets are currently skewed in the opposite direction. We lean more to meals made up of a ratio of 2% nutrient-filled, easily assimilated plant life to 98% acid-generating, stress-producing, high-protein foods.

The crux of this book is to show you that common everyday foods like bread, cereal, fish, chicken, and meat affect the acid level of your body, and the acid level of your body affects your health. Acidity and alkalinity are measured in terms of pH. Your internal systems operate in a slightly alkaline environment. We were designed to be slightly alkaline.

Acid that eventually gets inside your body where your cells are operating comes from food that is broken down in your digestive tract. Most digested foods leave a residue called ash. This ash is either acid, alkaline, or neutral. High-protein foods like meat, that make up such a large portion of our diets, leave acid ash. Fruits and vegetables (with a few exceptions) leave alkaline ash.

By reducing the amount of high-protein, acid ash-producing foods, and at the same time increasing the amount of alkaline ash-producing foods, your internal environmental conditions become right for optimum health.

Recall the basic four food groups that are almost second nature to us as the cornerstones of a "good diet": meat, poultry and fish; dairy products and eggs; cereals and grains; fruits and vegetables. Most of us have been drilled throughout our lives on the importance of including a balance of each of these groups in our daily diets. Let's take a look at how they stack up as far as acid or alkaline ash is concerned.

Meats, Poultry, Fish	*Very Acid*
Dairy Products, Eggs	*Acid*
Cereals, Grains	*Acid*
Fruits, Vegetables	*Alkaline*

When we follow the advice instilled in us, our daily diets contain 75% acid ash foods and only 25% alkaline ash foods. Let's be realistic about it: fruits and vegetables rarely make up 25% of the daily diets of most Americans.

WELLNESS PRINCIPLE: *Ketchup and relish don't cut it as "vegetables."*

Most of the nutrition information you were taught in school or that you read in magazine articles has been (to put it charitably) misleading. Although we have been given the best scientifically acceptable information available, by following it, as a nation we are getting sicker. Unfortunately, misinformation about healthful foods is not the only problem. We are polluting the environment in which we and the food we are growing are trying to live. But that is a topic for another time. The purpose of this book is to give you new insight into health and how you can make a few minor adjustments in the way you eat to pack better health into your life.

Fortunately, authoritative sources are modifying their recommendations concerning the constituents of a healthful diet. More and more we are being told to cut down on the amount of meat and fried foods we eat. Unfortunately, the nutrition sleuths have nailed the wrong suspect. Fat is being named the nutritional bugaboo that causes health problems. The biggest problem with fat is the meat it's attached to. While dietary recommendations concerning animal products are moving in the right direction, the reasons given for reducing meat consumption still miss the critical factor—the acidifying effect of protein. For instance:

A recent issue of *Time* magazine outlined current dietary recommendations from a report by the National Research Council. The Council recommended limiting fats to thirty percent of your daily calorie intake, and cholesterol consumption to thirty percent. We are told to "emphasize fish, skinless poultry, lean meats and low- or non-fat dairy products, and cut back on fried and other fatty foods such as pastries, spreads and dressings." The basis for these recommendations seems to be that people who eat large quantities of foods containing fats and cholesterol have a greater risk of heart attacks. We are told that plaque builds up in the arteries of people who eat a lot of meat and fried foods. It follows, then, that if you eat less fats, plaque and cholesterol will be kept under control; you won't be as likely to have a heart attack or stroke; and you probably won't be as prone to other diseases.

Very true, as far as the explanations go. However, there is much more to it than that. It's the acidifying effect from high fat and cholesterol foods that is the food culprit. Switching from "fatty" meats to "lean" meats isn't the whole answer. You may reduce the amount of fat you get, but fats leave a neutral ash. Lean meats leave proportionately more acid ash than fatty meats because the concentration of the acid ash producing parts is higher.

We are also told to increase consumption of vegetables and fruits. We aren't told why, other than that those who do seem to be healthier than those who don't. After you have read the chapters to come, you will understand the "why" of eating more fruits and vegetables. You will see that fruits and vegetables supply organic sodium that replenishes your alkaline reserve and keeps your internal environment slightly alkaline.

WELLNESS PRINCIPLE: *As your alkaline reserve goes, so goes your health.*

The greatest threat to your alkaline reserve is excess protein. You can survive and be healthy on considerably less protein than you are probably eating now. The 1980 Revised Recommended Daily Dietary Allowances (Food and Nutrition Board, National Academy of Sciences—National Research Council) suggests 56 grams of protein for adult males and 44 grams for most adult females. Yet the study I refer to in the chapter on osteoporosis shows that more calcium was lost than consumed each day when male subjects were on diets of only 47 grams of protein daily. Since most Americans eat more than 47 grams of protein a day, they are losing more calcium than they are taking in. When you understand the relationship between excess protein and physiological calcium levels, it isn't surprising that osteoporosis is a major health concern.

Throughout this book I caution you about changing your diet too quickly, even when you are changing for the better. I can't emphasize this enough. For your body to adjust to processing newly instituted foods takes time. Your body is supremely intelligent. It can adapt to just about any new conditions you inflict upon it, but it takes time. Quick adaptations are possible. However, they frequently excite unpleasant symptoms. If you have ever traveled outside the country and suffered from "Montezuma's Revenge," you have experienced one breed of quick-change symptoms. If you turn your food consumption patterns upside down by leaping with unrestrained enthusiasm into a new health-generating diet regimen, your health will improve quickly, but you'll feel worse in the process.

You may have tried a program similar to the one I propose, only to have met with semi-disastrous results. After a few days or a week, you may have experienced any of a number of unpleasant symptoms: lack of energy, diarrhea, headaches, or a general feeling of "yuck." You can suffer through all of these symptoms, and more, if you change your diet too fast. It's easy—but incorrect—to conclude from such a reaction that your new improved eating leads to misery, not health.

WELLNESS PRINCIPLE: *How you're feeling is not your best yardstick of health.*

You can eat your way to better health. Obviously, from the amount of money Americans spend on medical care each year, there is a basic problem with health in this country. We live better and have a more plentiful supply of food than most of the rest of the world. Yet too many of us, young and old alike, are sick. The unseemly high incidence of illness is reflected in the amount of money we spend on trying to feel better. The people of this nation are spending about $500 billion a year trying to ease the symptoms that result from eating too much of the types of foods that overstress their bodies.

Medical techniques can go only so far in curing ills. If we are to improve our individual or collective physical conditions, we must be aware of how various facets of our lifestyles can contribute to ill health. Food selection and tastes are major elements of lifestyle. Lifestyles can be improved.

STEPPING UP TO BETTER HEALTH

It's just as easy to be healthy as it is to be sick. Just give your body a chance by giving it the kind of foods that it works with best.

THE FIRST STEP to better health is to increase the amount of cooked vegetables you eat every day. For many people, one serving a day of any vegetable is a dramatic increase.

THE SECOND STEP is to reduce the amount of protein foods you eat each day. Have smaller servings of beef, poultry, or fish as you continue to add more cooked vegetables to your meals.

THE THIRD STEP is to cook the vegetables less and include one serving of raw vegetables or fruit every day.

THE FOURTH STEP is to begin to reduce your intake of salt, coffee, tea, cola drinks, and processed (fabricated) snack foods.

How fast can you make these changes? How fast is too fast? To answer these questions, we should understand the goal we are shooting for. *Ideally*, your daily diet (other than Thanksgiving, the Fourth of July, your birthday, and a limited assortment of other special occasions) should consist of a combination of:

45% cooked fruits and vegetables
30% raw fruits and vegetables
25% grains, nuts, seeds, meat, fish, or poultry

Since each of us follows his own individual eating pattern, the guidelines that follow are very general. The time frames suggested are for those who have been living on a diet of meats, "fast foods," processed or prepared ready-made foods, refined carbohydrates, and stimulants such as coffee, tea, cola, or alcoholic drinks. You may have been following a more healthful diet that already includes fresh, whole foods such as vegetables and fruits. If you have, you may be able to telescope the time periods recommended to suit your own health level. If your body has suffered food abuse for many years, you may need to extend each period. How your body responds is the best indicator of how fast you can improve your diet. No matter how fast you go, if unpleasant symptoms begin to appear (we'll talk later in the book about why this happens), back off. Reinstitute some of the foods your body is accustomed to, then again slowly eliminate them from your diet.

The next logical question is, "Are the recommended quantities by caloric value, bulk, or serving?" My answer: "Yes." No matter how you calculate it, *ideally* your menu items should be broken down into the 45%, 30%, and 25% proportions.

That is the Ideal Diet: 45% cooked vegetables and fruit, 30% raw vegetables and fruit, and 25% whatever else you want—meat, ice cream, chocolate cake, or any other favorite. This pattern is radically different from the way most of us now eat. You can expect to improve your diet and health for six months to a year or more before you even consider trying the Ideal Diet. For those who have been catering to their taste buds rather than to their bodies' needs, slow and steady movement toward better health is realistic.

SAMPLE TIMETABLE FOR IMPROVING YOUR DIET

To Begin	Add whole foods and cooked vegetables
After 3 or 4 Days	Add a serving of fruit
2 Weeks into the Program	Have one meal a day of fruit and cooked vegetables only
	Begin decreasing the amount of health inhibitors you consume (coffee, tea, cola drinks)

3 Weeks into the Program	Begin reducing salt Increase the amount of cooked vegetables and raw fruits
After the 1st Month	Begin reducing the amount of high protein foods
	Reduce intake of one health inhibitor each week (alcohol, cigarettes, chocolate, . . .)
	Begin adding "lightly" cooked or raw vegetables
Thereafter	Continue to increase amount of alkaline ash foods and decrease the amount of acid ash foods (Listed in Chapter 8)

These are general guidelines for improving your health. There is a more specific method of determining when your body is ready for the next step in good food—your morning urine pH values. In Chapter 10 is a more detailed explanation of the urine pH testing you read about (and, I hope, followed) at the beginning of this book. Later chapters give a more comprehensive method of evaluating your physiological acid level and health. Using the more detailed monitoring method, you can coordinate your diet changes with the rise and fall in morning urine pH values.

If your internal system isn't accustomed to coping with vegetables and fruit, don't shock it with a two-day flood of salads, raw broccoli, carrots, cucumbers, apples, bananas, and oranges. Take my word for it—violate this commandment and you'll pay for it. You will (a) develop diarrhea, muscle cramps, or headaches; (b) be nauseated or tired; (c) become short-tempered or depressed; or (d) all of the above.

There is one exception to the slow-and-steady rule: those who have a life-threatening disease and a highly alkaline morning urine pH of 8.0 after eating protein the night before. Anyone who fits into this category and wants to improve his health should have *only* raw foods. Raw celery, raw carrots, raw fruit, and freshly prepared raw vegetable and fruit juices. Nothing else. Certainly, he or she will lose weight and become weak on a raw fruit and vegetable diet. However, after sticking to this extreme for a while, the morning urine pH will begin to fall. It will ultimately drop as low as 5.5 pH. Three months of this extreme diet may be required before the pH begins to rise again. This is a severe crisis regimen to meet only a crisis situation.

If you are not in the "seriously ill" category but your morning urine test turned the pH paper a dark color after an acid ash meal the night before, you can begin your journey to health by adding some whole foods to your present menu. Whole brown rice, whole wheat, and cooked vegetables are good whole foods to add.

After three or four days of "conditioning" your body by adding whole foods and additional cooked vegetables to your normal menu, you can add even more vegetables and some fruit.

When you have been on the program for two weeks, it's time to start having one meal a day that is exclusively vegetables or fruit. During this phase, you will fare better if the vegetables are cooked the way you usually cook them.

You can now also begin to reduce slowly the amount of health inhibitors you put into your body. For example, start cutting down on the amount of coffee, tea, or cola drinks one week. The next week begin reducing salt. Then in weekly increments work on restricting sugar, alcohol, and cigarettes. The particular order you attack health inhibitors is of small consequence; you're working toward a long-term goal.

You may *temporarily* need supplements of pancreatic and plant enzymes to boost your vitality until your body can readapt to the unfamiliar nutritious foods. Enzymes are not absorbed, whether they be enzymes contained in whole foods or enzyme supplements. The end-products brought about by the work of the enzymes are absorbed. Short-term supplementation of enzymes helps your body to handle foods efficiently. After you have built up enough enzymes from whole foods, you won't need supplements.

The entry stage of diet modification is not the time to go "cold turkey" and cut out all red meat, dairy products, coffee, and soft drinks. Stifle your enthusiasm for speed. If it took twenty, thirty, or forty years of your body constantly adapting its physiological functions to get in the condition it's in now, it will take a while for it to retrace its steps to become accustomed to the kind of food designed for it.

Some vegetarians are able to start at the *2 Weeks into the Program* phase. Vegetarians who eat more vegetables and fruits than eggs and grains may be able to move toward the 75% alkaline: 25% acid ratio immediately and feel fine. Their metabolic processes are already geared to handling the kinds of foods their bodies need.

Folks who normally eat a lot of vegetables usually escape the quick-change blues even when they jump wholeheartedly into this program. One lady, despite multiple cautions, suddenly increased her intake of vegetables dramatically, and eliminated high-protein foods completely. She is in her mid-50s and had been a vegetable/fruit enthusiast for years. Her normal diet was better than most people's, although she ate some meat, eggs, dairy products, and a lot of grains, and drank a couple of cups of coffee a day.

Her chief complaint was that she felt "physically and mentally wrung out." She was "bloated," "mentally lethargic," and had no energy for her customary pleasures of racquetball and recreational walking. "I didn't know why I felt so bad," she commented. "I thought I was doing everything right."

She reasoned that since she already felt terrible, a quick change of diet couldn't make her feel much worse. So she acted on her standard premise: "If a little is good for you, a lot must be better." She charged headlong into more raw fruits, vegetables, and juices, cut out cereals and flesh foods, and throttled back on her coffee consumption. Her new way of eating bordered on Ideal.

Despite the crash change, within a few days both her energy level and enthusiasm soared. The bloated feeling disappeared as her body cleansed. She admitted to spending a lot of time in the bathroom as her body eliminated accumulated excess fluid.

This lady experienced a normal response for someone who has been diligent about keeping her alkaline reserve well stocked, even if she hadn't previously recognized the reason vegetables and fruits are prime contributors to health. She felt better almost immediately because her body was already accustomed to processing vegetables and fruits. Her major change was to avoid acid ash-producing foods altogether and add even more alkaline ash contributors.

Vegetarians can't necessarily expect such rapid changes just because they eat little or no meat. Those who eat a lot of acid ash-producing cereals and grains can suffer the same toxicity problems as meat eaters. Their big push should be to reduce substantially the amount of organic acid ash-producers they eat. They should cut way back on grains and cereals. Vegetarians too, should shoot for the 75% alkaline ash: 25% acid ash ratio in their daily diets.

Most people in the U.S. are on a more culturally typical diet—bacon and eggs, meat, and cheese. If you are either a grain eater or a meat eater still free of major illness, and your morning urine pH is generally acid, very likely you are healthy enough to reach the mostly-fruits-and-vegetables level in about six weeks. You can compress the conditioning time by beginning your eating day with fruit and increasing the amount of vegetables at other meals. Once you've started to break out in health, the first thing in your stomach should be fruit. It makes no difference if your first meal is at 5:00 A.M. or 2:00 P.M.—fruit first.

Anyone who has had his gallbladder removed should be particularly diligent about improving his diet. Removing an organ doesn't improve health. It may reduce symptoms, but it doesn't cure the underlying cause that brought about the symptoms in the first place. Those who must have their gallbladder removed are sick. Unless they change the conditions that brought about the problem, they are still sick after the gallbladder and pain are gone. Other symptoms will crop up elsewhere later. Gallbladder disease is a symptom of overall physiological distress. The problem is the person's health, not whether or not he has a gallbladder.

Although most of us aren't ready to undertake the Ideal Diet right off the bat, the response the quick-change lady experienced is to be expected by those who have knowingly or unknowingly kept their bodies slightly alkaline. It may take longer for most of us to reach the stage of being able to handle a diet made up principally of fruits and vegetables, but it can be done, and the rewards are well worth the dedication. How soon you get there depends upon several factors: your condition when you start; how long you deliberate before you get around to starting; and your motivation and dedication.

Remember, we eat to satisfy different needs. If eating acts as stress therapy for you, you may find it difficult to maintain your resolve to improve your health by eating better. The food you eat to feed an emotional need can have greater physiological effects on your body than food you eat just to sustain life. When your appetite is sparked by emotional stimuli, you have the double whammy of stressful thoughts generating physiological reactions which in turn can lead you to revert to your habitual eating patterns rather quickly. If this happens and you feel guilty about it, you will be doing your body more harm than if you didn't try the improvements at all.

The key to dietary change, regardless of where you start, is how you feel. If you begin to feel bad and develop symptoms such as diarrhea, excessive fatigue, or headaches, you're changing too fast. You're getting better, but you need to slow down. Your body won't be hurt, but your commitment to change will self-destruct.

Again, under Ideal conditions, six months to a year may be required before your body functions normally again. This program isn't a quick-fix fad diet. It's the beginning of an eating style that can carry you along the road to a lifetime of health. Your objective is to be healthy and pain-free as long as you live. Old age is no excuse for disease. We're all going to die sometime, but there's no law that says you have to get sicker along the way. You may as well be healthy as long as you live.

CHAPTER 7

The Power of Change

Throughout this book, I repeat the warning, "Do not change your diet too quickly." The "failure" of many effective, health-enhancing diet programs is probably due more to the unpleasant aftermath of rapid diet change than to anything else. Several excellent weight-loss and health-oriented nutrition plans that could improve health have been in vogue in the past few years. Unfortunately, most of them fade from the limelight and general use because of improper implementation. Enthusiasm gives way to discomfort as many people leap into diet changes too quickly. After a few weeks on their new programs, they begin to feel worse than they did before they started. Health-seeking dieters come to the conclusion that if this is how it feels to be healthier, they'd rather not.

The story of one of my patients is an excellent example of how a dramatic, sudden turn to a good diet can call into question the wisdom of continuing a new eating program.

Barry and I had known each other through business for several years. (Of course, "Barry" isn't his real name, but the person and the story are real.) Although Barry had been to my clinic on business many times, he had never been there as a patient. This story began on Super Bowl Sunday. My phone rang during the game. The interruption was probably the most exciting part of this particular gridiron contest. When I answered, Barry identified himself and followed quickly with "I need your help."

44

Barry gave me a quick sketch of his physical problems. In a nutshell, he had been having extremely severe allergic reactions for about three weeks. The allergens that were keeping him in a state of near panic fell into three categories—food, water, and air. You can't get much more fundamental than that.

Barry had been to several other doctors about his problem: his family doctor, allergy specialists, and an environmental allergy clinic. He had been treated, experienced temporary relief, and been told that he would be out of work for about a year.

On the Sunday he telephoned, he was having another severe reaction. Nothing he did relieved his symptoms. His chief complaints were that he was having trouble breathing and that his muscles were twitching uncontrollably. He had followed his doctors' instructions to the letter. He had isolated himself in one "allergy-free" room of his home and had the heat duct to that room closed off. He was so sensitive to everything, he couldn't even tolerate the air from the furnace. And he was getting worse. I knew from his description of his condition and lifestyle that he couldn't tolerate the environment of a public building like my clinic either. I realized that he was suffering from all of the three T's—Timing, Toxicity, and Thoughts. So I arranged to see him at his house the first thing the next morning.

Early Monday morning, I treated him at his home. I also extracted from him a commitment that he would attend my week of Concentrated Care that was coming up the following week, and told him to be at the clinic at 9:00 A.M. the next day. On my way home from the clinic that evening, I checked in on him. He met me at the door, smiling.

Barry showed up on Tuesday as instructed. He was feeling much better and was breathing more easily. During his first visit to the clinic as a patient, I treated him and told him what foods he should and should not eat if he wanted to get better and stay better. In essence, I told him, "No meat and lots of fruits and vegetables." Cutting down on meat wasn't much of a problem for him. He didn't feel well enough to eat much. For several weeks, he hadn't been able to eat anything except green beans, zucchini, and filtered water. He had lost about twenty pounds and looked almost gaunt. Barry was sick.

One or two treatments had substantially corrected his Timing and Thoughts problems. That was no big deal. He was then able to begin eating some fruit and some vegetables other than green beans and zucchini. On Wednesday of that week, about 340 days short of his year out of work, he went back to his office for a short time "to check the mail." The following week, he attended the Concentrated Care program in a group of about thirty people.

Keep in mind that this man hadn't been able to go anyplace or be away from his "environmentally controlled" surroundings without suffering extreme distress. Aromas that are common in groups of people—shaving lotion, hand lotion, hair spray and the like—had recently brought on violent reactions. But here he was in a closed room with about thirty people who had no idea that their personal grooming habits might cause Barry major discomfort.

The treatments he had received the week before the Concentrated Care program had improved his Timing and cleared his Thoughts problem enough to allow him to venture farther from the sanctuary of his room. With that done, he could again join the world. However, in order to continue to improve, he had to be conscientious about his diet.

Barry was extremely ill. He had to make swift and sure adjustments to his diet. To climb back on the road to health, he had to do just what I have been telling you not to do. He had to change his diet radically and quickly. I would like to be able to report that once he started to improve he has felt fantastic ever since. However, that is not the case. He has had his ups and downs, but more ups than downs; and the downs can't compare with how down he was when he was ill. He is back at work full-time now. Back in the same world in which he lived and worked while he was getting sick. Now, however, he knows how to handle stress and frustrations better; he comes to the clinic periodically for treatment; and he is much more aware of how food affects his body and his attitudes. He is greatly improved but not completely recovered, yet.

WELLNESS PRINCIPLE: *Feeling good and being healthy aren't necessarily synonymous.*

About three months after his major crisis, Barry came in for one of his regular treatments. He wasn't feeling very good. However, this time it wasn't because he was getting sick. It was because he was getting well.

Barry described his symptoms. "On Sundays, I feel pretty good; but on Mondays, I go back to work and I'm in trouble again."

With this brief description of the way he felt, I could fill in the gaps. I elaborated what he was saying.

"You feel 'scattered.' You can't focus on a thought and carry it through. You get a thought, and before you can finish that thought, three other thoughts have jumped into your mind. You're not congruent. You're not centered. You're everywhere all the time."

"That's it," agreed Barry. "That's just how I feel."

His symptoms were the result of his quick diet change. In the beginning, I had told him to eat lots of fruit, and the fruit made him feel better. It was restocking his alkaline reserve and giving his body a chance to function more normally. Yet, after a couple of months of a heavy concentration of fruit, the more fruit he ate, the worse he felt. Fruit had made him feel good at first, so he ate even more of it in an effort to feel good again. He was, indeed, getting better by eating the fruit, but he was feeling worse.

To understand how he could feel as bad as he did while he was gaining in health, we need to know a little about his nutrition background.

Before he became obviously ill, Barry had followed the conventional diet similar to that of most Americans. In fact, he admitted to some dietary habits that top many people's as far as being self-destructive. He told me that he "always" had a cola drink near at hand. He generally drank about three or four cola drinks a day. In addition, he was what he described as a "candy bar and pasta nut." Carbonated cola, candy bars, and pasta were among the major contributors to his illness. Barry's body was exhausted from coping with improper food.

After years of dietary abuse, his body was running exclusively on backup systems to handle the non-stop toxic substances that he poured in. His allergic reactions were responses of exhausted adrenal glands and other physiologic systems. As a result, his body was in severe defense. It was surviving by functioning on backup systems. The allergic reactions were his body's way of telling him that he had imposed too many stresses on it. It was coping, but just barely.

In addition, Barry was extremely anxious—actually fear-ridden. When I saw him that first Monday, he was, in his words, "living from hour to hour." His mind was racing with apprehension. "Why me?" He was in his early 40s. He had a wife and two children to support. He couldn't work. He couldn't eat the way he usually did. He couldn't drink the water from the tap in his own home. He couldn't breathe the air that circulated in his home. He couldn't even take a shower unless the water was filtered through charcoal before it touched his body. "Why me?"

As he was helped over the initial hurdle of his illness, Barry began to improve his diet. He eliminated animal protein from his meals and ate mostly fruits and vegetables. This regimen has a cleansing effect on the body. It allows accumulated toxins to be eliminated so the body can get on with healing itself. With all of the fruit he was eating, his body began a process of internal cleansing, and he felt better. After a while, he added a little bit of fish, then a little bit of chicken and turkey. Then two things happened.

First, his body was cleaning out toxins faster than his elimination systems could get rid of them. He was cleansing too fast.

To counteract this, I told him to eat some beef—a steak or hamburger, or whatever suited his fancy. Although I had told him previously that meat stresses his body, he followed my advice and ate a hamburger. The next day, he reported that he felt much better.

Why would eating a hamburger make him feel better? It certainly wasn't making him healthier. If beef were a health producer, most Americans wouldn't have even a millisecond of illness.

Barry's hamburger made him feel better because it slowed his body's cleansing process. His improved diet had allowed his body to begin to clear out some of the toxins that had been accumulating over the years. However, as soon as that mouth-watering, cholesterol-filled, grease-dripping hamburger entered his stomach, Barry's body stopped cleaning out the toxins from previous candy bars, colas, and hamburgers and attended to the newly introduced heavy-duty substances. Cleansing stopped while more pressing business was conducted.

Cleansing is a healing process; and healing can't take place while the body is trying to survive.

This is why a constant diet of foods that stress your body leads to disease. Your natural healing ability can't function while your body is geared to meet an emergency.

WELLNESS PRINCIPLE: *Eating improper food sparks a physiological emergency.*

The second effect of Barry's quick diet change was that his circumstances outstripped his beliefs.

He was obviously better than he had been; he was back at work. He had believed the doctors who had told him only a couple of months earlier that he wouldn't be able to work for a year. Yet, he was working. Reality didn't match his beliefs.

We know that the body is an integrated unit. Everything that affects the physiology affects the mind; and everything that affects the mind affects the physiology. Barry's mind-body connection was contributing to his feeling bad although he was getting healthier.

Barry's improved diet was allowing his body to take care of his toxicity problem. However, the large amounts of fruit he was eating began to affect his Thoughts. The fruit was having an expansive effect on him. *He* wasn't expanding, his thought processes were. As we see in Chapter 21, particular types of foods affect our thoughts and personalities in particular ways. Fruits and vegetables have an expansive effect. *Expansive* might best be illustrated by the drug culture term of the '60s—*mind expanding.* Too much of a mind-expanding substance, even health-producing fruit and fruit juice, can take you off to a mental never-never land. Concentration is almost impossible. Focusing on a single thought is almost impossible.

On the other hand, beef and other meat has a contractive effect. It prompts the body to focus more inwardly to tighten things down. In Barry's case, the contractive effect of the hamburger offset some of the expansive effect of the fruit. It brought him "back down to earth."

So Barry's hamburger affected his physiology and his thoughts. It also had a psychological effect on him. Eating that hamburger told him that he can eat anything he wants. He isn't sick any more. There is nothing wrong with him. He is recovering. His body is in high gear for healing. If he can eat what he wants, he can also work, despite having been told he wouldn't be able to for a year.

Let's look at the situation from Barry's point of view:

A specialist told him he would be out of work for a year. Barry believed what he had been told. He had confidence in the doctor.

Implication: *there is something seriously wrong with you.*

Then I told him that he could go back to work.

Implication: *there's nothing wrong with you.*

But I also told him that he had to eat certain types of foods and not eat certain other types of foods.

Implication: *there's something wrong with you or you could eat anything you want.*

Now, I tell Barry, "Go eat a hamburger or steak."

Implication: *there's nothing wrong with you.*

Barry was receiving mixed signals. This is why he was "getting into trouble" when he went to work. His subconscious mind was still functioning on the premise that he was sick and couldn't work. Consequently, when he went to work, he felt bad.

He knew that he needed fruits and vegetables to continue to improve, but when he ate the hamburger, a "forbidden" food, there were no serious repercussions. He can, indeed, eat anything he wants. He isn't sick. Finally, belief, perception, and reality are synchronized.

The purpose of the story of Barry is to emphasize the importance of changing your eating habits in an orderly fashion. (You probably also picked up on the crucial role that Thoughts, particularly negative Thoughts like "you won't be able to work for a year," play in your health.)

Feeling worse after changing to a more healthful way of eating has caused many people to abandon their goal of improving their health by improving their diets. I can't stress enough that if you change your eating habits for the better too quickly, your body will begin its internal housecleaning as though it were spring cleaning time at Tara. Everything that needs to go, goes. You will feel better for a while, then you will feel worse than you did before you started.

Barry was a prime example of this. Before he became ill, he followed the conventional basic-four diet. When he came to me, I told him to eat plenty of fruits and vegetables. Then, after a while, his body's responses indicated that he could add a little bit of fish, then a little bit of chicken and turkey. Being heavy into fruits and vegetables and light on processed food was a radical departure from the fare his body had been accustomed to handling. His body began to clean up its act. But it happened very fast.

In addition to feeling better and being able to eat, drink water from the tap, and breathe easily again, Barry went back to work. Yet he had been told by someone he believed in that he wouldn't be able to work for a year. His belief and his actions were in conflict. Any time we act in a way that is contrary to our beliefs, we subject ourselves to inner turmoil.

Barry's story illustrates that you can change your actions quickly. And you can change your diet quickly. However, when you change the substances that go into your body, it will respond differently than before. The nutrients from food are used to replenish and repair cells. Cells make up your body. Components of that food ultimately becomes part of you. The substances that go into your body become the materials of your body. You can't change what your body is made of instantly without noticeable effects.

Similarly, quick changes in attitudes and perceptions may cause you distress. Your actions are based on your beliefs. Your beliefs are based on your past experiences. Barry "believed" that he was sick and couldn't work. It wasn't until he ate that fateful hamburger that his belief in his illness gave way to belief in his health. You can change your beliefs, but in the process, it causes you to look at yourself and the world in a different light.

Remember, you are an integrated being: body and mind are as closely related as cell and nucleus. Events and ingredients that affect one affect the other. You must take both into consideration whenever you change any part of your lifestyle, including diet.

CHAPTER 8

Acid Should Run Batteries, Not Bodies

As you read these words, you are generating acid. Not only are you generating acid, you are eliminating it. But, not to worry. You're not flaunting any rules of etiquette; everyone does it all the time. However, to put you at ease, I'll explain. Your cells produce acid as they function, and your lungs eliminate it every time you exhale. All is well and good.

Your body must constantly contend with acid. The acid your body produces is relatively weak and usually doesn't cause any problems. On the other hand, the acid you get from eating too much protein and other acid-producing foods is stronger, and it causes lots of problems. The concept that the acid level of the body may be a major factor of health started to become apparent to me over a decade ago when I was catapulted into the study of nutrition.

Learning as much as I could about how food affects the body hadn't been one of my original life-goals. Yet, experience was showing me that if I was going to fulfill my professional goal of helping sick people get well, I needed to know more about the relationship between food and total health.

I had accumulated conclusive clinical evidence that diet had a profound effect on how well and how quickly patients responded to my treatments. I found that my efforts to help patients improve were analogous to getting an engine into top running form. I could adjust the mechanical and electrical systems and get the parts working correctly, but sometimes the engine would run only falteringly. If after I had tuned the engine the owner put the wrong kind of fuel in the tank, the well-tuned engine could be ruined.

> **WELLNESS PRINCIPLE:** *A well-tuned body doesn't run well on inferior fuel.*

So I began what has become a continuous investigation into nutrition and the relationship between food and health. As I poured over textbooks of the various scientific disciplines, I found that the subject of pH kept reappearing. I read about enzymes and ran into pH; I pondered protein and there was pH. Technical explanations describing the production and operation of blood, liver, interstitial fluid, intracellular fluid, urine, saliva, and all the fluids of the body brought up pH.

The term pH stands for "potential of Hydrogen"—it's a measure of the relative acidity or alkalinity of a solution.

Acid comes in different degrees of potency. You eat citric acid in fruits with no ill effect; but the hydrochloric acid in the chemistry lab can drill a hole through flesh and other less sensitive substances. Although there is more to determining the potency of acids than just pH, for our purpose of investigating the effects of various foods, pH is the major factor.

The pH of a substance is measured on a scale from 0.00 to 14.00. The midpoint, 7.00, is neutral: it is neither alkaline nor acid. Water (assuming it is reasonably unpolluted) has a pH of 7.0. The lower the number, the more acidic the solution; the higher the number, the more alkaline the solution. A very general "picture" of the pH scale looks like the diagram shown on the next page.

You will see from this scale that a pH of 8 is slightly alkaline, while a pH of 12 is very alkaline; a pH of 6 is slightly acid, and a pH of 2 is very acid. The pH of body fluids is measured more precisely than by whole numbers; it is usually shown in tenths or hundredths, such as 6.2 or 7.35. In the world of pH, there is a vast difference between two consecutive whole pH numbers. A brief elaboration of the basics of pH may be helpful.

pH SCALE OF ACIDIC REACTION				N E U T R A L	ALKALINE			
ACID					ALKALINE			
Total	Very	Moderate	Slight		Slight	Moderate	Very	Total
0	1 2	3 4	5 6	7	8 9	10 11	12 13	14

Since pH values represent a logarithmic scale, there is a tenfold difference between each unit. For instance, pH 5.0 is ten times more acid than pH 6.0, but pH 4.0 is one hundred times (10 x 10) more acid than pH 6.0. So you can see that minor variations in the tenths or hundredths are more significant than might appear at first glance—much more significant, certainly, than tenths or hundredths of a dollar these days. The difference between 7.25 and 7.40 pH of blood is considerably more impressive than the difference between $7.25 and $7.40 for a meal. Small changes in pH readings represent major changes in the way your body functions.

WELLNESS PRINCIPLE: *pH indicates acidity or alkalinity AND how healthy you are.*

The pH of the fluids in your body doesn't stay constant; it fluctuates according to what's going on. If it fluctuates too widely or for too long, you encounter physical problems. As I became engrossed in studying nutrition, one of the things that I found baffling was the vast range that was given as "normal" for the pH of certain body fluids. Some fluids, such as blood, had a very narrow range (7.35 to 7.45); others, like gallbladder bile (5.50 to 7.70) or the substances in the duodenum (4.20 to 8.20), had great gulfs between their outer limits of "normal."

Since there is such a dramatic difference between pH 4.20 (which is relatively acidic for the body) and pH 8.20 (which is quite alkaline for the body), I was perplexed by the intelligent body doing something that appeared to be inconsistent. A statement I read in a physiology text added to the mystery: "Only slight changes in hydrogen ion concentration [pH] from the normal value can cause marked alterations in the rates of chemical reactions in the cells,..."[1] If slight changes in intracellular pH can cause decided changes in cellular reactions, why would it be necessary for the pH of a particular extracellular fluid to fluctuate so widely? Take a look at some of the "normals" given for substances in your body, keeping in mind that 6.0 is ten times more acid than 7.0, and that 5.0 is one hundred times more acid than 7.0. These are more than "slight changes."

pH Normals[2,3,4] (Extracellular)	
Blood	7.35 - 7.45
Spinal Fluid	7.30 - 7.50
Saliva	6.50 - 7.50
Gastric	1.00 - 3.50
Duodenum	4.20 - 8.20
Feces	4.60 - 8.40
Urine	4.80 - 8.40
Liver Bile	7.10 - 8.50
Gall Bladder Bile	5.50 - 7.70
Pancreas	8.00 - 8.30

All of the fluids of the body, with the exception of those in the stomach, are—or can be—alkaline. To refresh your memory about the difference between alkaline and acid, bicarbonate of soda is alkaline; it can neutralize the burning effects of strong acids. Vinegar is acid; it can neutralize the corrosive effects of very strong alkalis. Both strong acids and strong alkalis can damage tissue and cause pain. The alkaline substances inherent in the body are weak; some of the acids produced as a result of different foods we eat are relatively strong.

WELLNESS PRINCIPLE: *Your body is an alkaline entity by design . . .*

It's important to understand that all of the body fluids, except those in the stomach, are alkaline. To simplify matters, we will establish now that fluids in the stomach are inherently acid. (When I refer to "body fluids," I am talking about all fluids with the exception of those in the stomach.)

There's a lot of fluid in your body: blood, bile, pancreatic juice, gastrointestinal fluid, cerebrospinal fluid, synovial fluid, saliva, urine, aqueous humor, and others. The average-size adult's body sloshes about with nearly forty-two quarts of fluid. There is fluid inside the cells, outside the cells, as part of the blood, around the joints, in and around the brain and spinal cord, and in and around organs. All fluid is supposed to be alkaline. That is, it should register above 7.0 on the pH scale.

So, here we are with a body that is filled with over ten gallons of fluid, most of which *should* be alkaline, yet some very vital organs are housing or producing very acidic substances. We can understand the gastric juice of the stomach at pH 1.00 to pH 3.50; strong acids can break down some pretty tough substances for digestion. But the wide variation in the range of the pH of some other fluids didn't seem logical.

The wide pH ranges occur in fluids that leave the body. To me, this indicates that the body responds to different stresses or types of foods in a manner that would maintain a very narrow pH range inside the cells. What would cause the urine to range from a rather acidic pH 4.8 to a rather alkaline pH 8.4? Of more importance, why would this fluctuation be necessary?

WELLNESS PRINCIPLE: *Your body is alkaline by design and acid producing by function.*

Obviously, although your body is an alkaline entity, acid is not foreign to it. In fact, acid is produced at a good clip all the time. Cells operate in an alkaline environment, yet acid is produced as they function; and cells that are alive function all the time. However, this acid by itself won't damage your body because it is a weak acid that is easily eliminated by your lungs. This is why you huff and puff when you exercise vigorously. Your body is getting rid of the acid generated by hard-working cells.

The second source of acid is neither quite so innocuous nor easily taken care of—the acid from acid ash food. This acid is much stronger than the acid produced by cells and must be neutralized before it can be eliminated through the kidneys. If you eat the same kinds of food as most Americans, seventy-five percent to ninety-five percent of your daily diet consists of acid ash-producing food. Most food isn't acid when you eat it, but acid ash is left as it is processed. If most of the food you eat leaves strong, hard-to-handle acid ash, it's just a matter of time before your body becomes too acid. Excess acid from acid ash foods can be eliminated, but it can't be eliminated through the lungs. Dietary acid ash is eliminated through the kidneys. In the process, *vital minerals are lost with it.* Understanding this point is crucial to understanding how certain types of food are detrimental to your health and why you should be concerned about how much acid ash-producing foods you eat.

As pointed out in Chapter 6, foods in three of the four basic food groups are essentially acid producers. Of the "basic four" food groups, meats, dairy, fruits and vegetables, and grains, meats, dairy products, and grains are all acid ash-producing foods. Acid ash from these foods can be eliminated through the kidneys and bowels, but it must first be neutralized. It is neutralized by a process called buffering. If the acid weren't neutralized, it would burn sensitive tissue on its way through the digestive tract. See how smart your body is? Without thought on your part, it saves you pain and discomfort everyday.

Those who sometimes have pain or burning when they urinate may wonder if their internal intelligence has deserted them. It hasn't. Any system can be abused beyond its coping limits. Pain or burning on urination is an indicator that the reserves of neutralizing minerals are exhausted and that the body has adapted the way it functions for survival, not comfort. Pain on urination can usually be alleviated by drinking several glasses of cranberry juice a day for a few days. This won't affect the underlying cause of the pain, but it will ease the symptoms. The sufferer will be more comfortable, but he will continue to get sicker unless he changes his ways to correct the cause. The only way to improve the condition that caused the problem is to eat foods that will replenish the supply of neutralizing minerals—the alkaline reserve.

WELLNESS PRINCIPLE: *You can never eliminate enough symptoms to correct the problem that is the cause of the symptoms.*

Your first line of defense against the damaging effects of dietary acid ash is your alkaline reserve. If the acid ash produced by food isn't neutralized, your body will become so toxic that it can no longer function. (That's a euphemism for "If your body gets too acidic, you'll die.")

Your alkaline reserve is made up of minerals that offset the effects of dietary acid ash. The principal minerals are sodium, calcium, potassium, and magnesium. You get these in fruits and vegetables, not table salt and supplements. Minerals in granular form (such as table salt) or pill form (such as supplements) aren't the same as those that are packaged in Mother Nature's original containers—plants. Fruits and vegetables contain *organic* minerals; table salt and many supplements contain *inorganic* minerals.

The terms *organic* and *inorganic* will be used a lot as we progress. The way elements of a compound are connected determines whether it is organic or inorganic.

The elements of organic minerals are loosely held together; they are attracted to each other but are separable—like brother and sister.

The constituent parts of inorganic minerals are held together tightly; they have strong bonds that the body can't break easily. Sodium and chloride that make up table salt are attached by inorganic bonds; like teenagers and telephones, once together, they're hard to get apart.

We'll go into organic and inorganic bonds more thoroughly in another chapter. For now, *organic* = easily broken apart; *inorganic* = tightly held together.

Your body uses organic minerals to buffer (neutralize) dietary acid ash. The most important of these minerals is sodium. Neutralizing minerals are a part of your alkaline reserve. Most of the sodium used in buffering is stored in the liver and muscles ready to be used as needed. As with most materials used on demand, if the supply isn't replenished, eventually it will be depleted.

WELLNESS PRINCIPLE: *Health depends on adequate reserves of resources.*

Think of the minerals in your alkaline reserve as dollars in a cookie jar. You can take out all of the money at once and the jar will be empty right away, or you can take out a little each day and it will take longer to whittle down the store. Either way, if you don't put something back in, eventually your supply will be gone.

In the case of the sodium of your alkaline reserve, each time you eat protein and other foods that add acid ash to your body, some of the precious sodium from your stored reserve is used. If you don't replace it with the sodium from fruits and vegetables, your valuable reserve of alkaline minerals will vanish like marshmallows at a picnic. That doesn't mean you're going to wither up and die the minute your store of sodium is drained. Your body is at least as determined to keep going as you are. There are alternative sources of minerals, such as calcium, to neutralize acid ash from food, and you have a great source of calcium in your bones.

The problem with using calcium as a backup is that calcium is supposed to be doing something else. The principle job of calcium is to keep your bones "solid." When the calcium must be used to serve another purpose, its primary function is being shortchanged. Osteoporosis develops when your calcium has gone off to play hero and bail you out of the mess caused by your dietary habits. However, if that's what it takes to keep you alive, that's what will happen. You can live with crumbling bones, but you can't live if your body is too acid.

Now you are beginning to see why I went into all of that about the body being so intelligent; it adapts the function of one thing to take care of stresses put on it someplace else. One of the biggest unintentional stresses is produced when we eat more acid-producing foods than reserve-replenishing foods. Vegetables and fruits build up your reserve of organic minerals; acid-producing foods keep taking them out.

HEALTH HINT

You need adequate amounts of vegetables and fruits to take care of the acid that is produced by meats, fish, poultry, dairy products, seeds, nuts, and grains.

"But, what about all of the acid in fruits?" you may ask.

Good question. To be sure, if you put a piece of pH paper in the juice of a fresh lemon, orange, grapefruit, or even an apple, you will get an acid reading. Some fruits are so acid that the pH paper won't even turn color. Yet most fruits do not add to the acid ash level of your body. Only a few fruits are exceptions to this rule. Prunes, plums, and cranberries have an acidifying effect that has nothing to do with acidity of the fruits themselves, but rather with the type of acid they contain (aromatic). This type of acid is not changed to carbon dioxide in the body. It goes in acid and comes out acid.

Most fruit acid is organic and is easily processed and eliminated, and it leaves an alkaline ash. Organic acids are converted to weak carbonic acid in the body. Carbonic acid converts to carbon dioxide that is exhaled through the lungs. Not only is fruit easy on your body as far as acid is concerned, it also provides organic sodium to replenish your alkaline reserve. Fruits and vegetables go into your mouth acid but leave an alkaline ash to add to your alkaline reserve.

WELLNESS PRINCIPLE: *Fruits are acid entities that serve an alkalizing function.*

Food isn't the only thing that causes acid. We have said that as the cells function, acid is produced. The faster cells function, the more acid they generate.

This may appear to be a contradiction to our premise that the body never makes a mistake. If the body operates in an alkaline environment, why would cells make acid? Acid generated by the body is a by-product of energy production and is easily eliminated.

We operate at the cellular level. If the cells don't work, the body doesn't work. Like anything else that functions, cells must have energy.

You were probably told as a child that you needed to eat good, nutritional food to "keep up your energy." Very true. We get energy from food, but it isn't a direct process. It's not quite like pouring gasoline into the fuel tank of your car and having it pumped directly to the engine to burn. Energy from food is a special kind of energy that is generated through a more circuitous route from source to end.

For instance, take that hamburger with lettuce, pickles, onions, grated cheese, and special sauce on a sesame seed bun you had for lunch. Before any of that can turn into energy in the cells, the carbohydrates must be changed into glucose, the protein must be converted into amino acids, and the fats turned into fatty acids. When these usable materials get inside the cells, they react with oxygen and various enzymes to release energy that is used to form adenosine triphosphate (ATP). This reaction takes place in little energy factories inside the cell called mitochondria. It's the ATP produced inside the cell that is used to provide the special energy for metabolic activity, and it's all that energy-producing activity inside the cell that produces acid. The only cells that don't have the capability of producing acids are mature red blood cells; they lose their mitochondria as they mature. The acid the body makes is a by-product of cellular respiration—mainly aerobic respiration. *Aerobic* means "with oxygen." We're all familiar with aerobic exercises, such as jogging and calisthenics set to music, that are designed to make your heart beat faster, your lungs work harder, and your sweat glands go into overdrive. Aerobic activity involves a lot of oxygen and produces about ten times more acid than its wimp cousin, anaerobic activity.

Anaerobic means without oxygen. Weight lifting and isometric exercises can be considered anaerobic (but not wimpy) exercises. They involve strength and short bursts of activity that don't substantially increase the oxygen intake. Consequently, anaerobic exercise causes less acid to be generated than does aerobic exercise.

Even though cells generate acid as they produce energy, this acid is not a threat to the body. It can be eliminated through the lungs. Eliminating acid this way doesn't take any minerals from your alkaline reserve. This point is so crucial to understanding why the body can handle naturally produced acid yet must adapt to handle acid from acid ash-producing foods that it will be repeated in various places and contexts throughout this book.

It isn't the acid generated by cells that causes a problem; it's the excess acid that comes from eating more acid ash-producing foods than the body can process without altering its natural way of functioning.

> **WELLNESS PRINCIPLE:** *A health-sustaining diet is a matter of proportions.*

Perhaps a recap of the different types of acid your body must deal with will be helpful.

THREE SOURCES OF ACID

1. *Fruits*   Contain organic acid the body can eliminate through the lungs.

   Contribute to the alkaline reserve.

   Put little stress on the body.

2. *Cellular Activity*   Produces weak acid that can be eliminated through the lungs.

   Does not stress the body excessively.

3. *Acid-Producing Foods*   Leave strong acids.

   Must be neutralized before being eliminated through kidneys or colon.

   Are highly stressful to the body.

   Take minerals from the alkaline reserve.

The only time naturally produced acid may become a health threat is when acid from strenuous exercise tops off excess acid from food. Joggers, professional athletes, and others who exercise a lot are at risk if their systems have already reached the maximum tolerable limits of dietary acid build-up. If they are already acidotic, when they exercise, acid is generated faster than the body can get rid of it. If they can live long enough to pant, they'll survive. If they can't, they don't.

It may be only a matter of seconds between the time the exercise acid is formed and the time it can be eliminated through the lungs. But when the body is already overly acid and more acid of any kind is added, regardless of the source, it can be a fatal addition.

If a person has a big meal of food that has an acidifying effect, then goes out to exercise, this person can die. Acid on top of acid can raise the acid level to disastrous heights (which means it lowers the pH readings dramatically). Recall the extremely narrow range of tolerance for blood pH—7.35 to 7.45. The meal by itself won't kill him and the exercise by itself won't kill him; but the two combined can. That's why you should *never* exercise after a big meal.

WELLNESS PRINCIPLE: *Mind your manners—never eat and run.*

Understanding that exercise adds acid to the body takes some of the mystery out of why we frequently hear of athletes dying while working out or jogging.

I'm not opposed to exercise! But jogging and other strenuous exercise should never be used to "get healthy." You get healthy at the meal table first. When you are healthy, then you can jog or exercise to maintain your health and to build strength. Fitness and strength are not synonymous with health!

Many athletes and physical fitness buffs are high-protein enthusiasts. Protein creates a tremendous amount of acid—sometimes more than the heart can stand. If you are high on fitness and your body is high in acid, make sure you keep your heart rate under 120 beats per minute when you exercise. You can push your heart rate up again when your acid level goes down.

You are perfectly safe jogging, playing tennis, cross-country skiing, playing water polo, or shoveling snow as long as you put the proper fuel in your body. You need *more* alkalizing foods than acidifying. It's as simple as that.

There are real perils in eating too many foods that produce acid without offsetting them with enough foods to provide neutralizing minerals. When your body must fight to maintain life-sustaining pH levels, you are a prime candidate for progressive disease—or worse.

CHAPTER 9

A Cruise Down the Alimentary Canal

Join me on a journey. We'll use high-tech, state-of-the-art imagination to travel the route taken by our daily bread and other goodies. We are going to have an on-site look at how pH affects some very important physiological processes. To help us in our investigation, we'll take along a pH meter and a couple of reference books as travel guides.

We'll begin at the beginning of the digestive system—the mouth. This is a good place for our first pH reading; there is a lot of saliva in here. Our tour guide reference book says saliva is supposed to be between pH 6.50 and 7.50. But the pH meter is registering only 5.8. That's strange.

Saliva contains an enzyme called ptyalin. Its job is to break down large starch molecules into smaller units so they can be used farther down the road. Ptyalin works best around pH 6.5 or above. It isn't logical that the body would put an enzyme designed to function in an alkaline environment in an acidic environment of pH 5.8 and expect it to work. The body wouldn't create a substance and put it in an environment that hinders its functioning unless it had to.

If the environment had been designed to be acid, the enzymes would be the sort that would work best in an acid climate. Nature makes enzymes that work in more acid conditions. The saliva of dogs, for instance, ranges from pH 3.0 to 5.0. But dogs aren't basically starch-eaters; they are meat-eaters. Their saliva serves the same pre-digestion function as man's but is designed to work on tougher substances. Man's saliva was fashioned to prepare plant life for processing.

We haven't even progressed beyond the mouth and already a mystery has cropped up. We'll move on, and perhaps we'll find a solution.

With the help of peristaltic waves, we'll slide down the esophagus to the stomach. We'll have to wriggle through the stricture between the esophagus and stomach.

In the stomach we find an entirely different situation from that in the mouth. It's nasty! Our pH meter shows an extremely acid 2.00.

Gastric juices, including hydrochloric acid, are produced here. Hydrochloric acid is a strong acid secreted by cells of the wall of the stomach. We also find that the enzyme pepsin is being made from pepsinogen. Pepsin begins protein digestion in the stomach. The atmosphere here is good for pepsin to do its job. Pepsin works best at a pH of 2.00 to 3.00.[1]

WELLNESS PRINCIPLE: *If at all possible, the body always puts any substance it produces in a desirable environment.*

It's interesting to note that the food here in the stomach is stored and processed in layers; it's not all jumbled up and churning around, even though sometimes we feel as if it were. The food that arrived first is nearest the wall and is worked on first. Gastric glands in the wall of the stomach secrete the digestive juices to process the food.

There's not much more to see here and it's pretty unpleasant in this highly acid atmosphere. Let's continue.

We exit the stomach through the pylorus (sometimes called the pyloric valve) and emerge in the duodenum to encounter another dramatic change in climate. There is mucus everywhere! Lots of little cells of Brunner's glands all around the walls are spitting out mucus. There are a few enzymes here also, but mostly mucus. It appears that the pH climate of the duodenum depends on whether or not partially digested food called chyme (pronounced kime) is being pumped in from the stomach. When chyme is coming in, the environment is very acid; when there's no chyme, it's slightly alkaline.

As we move along the upper course of the small intestine, we see an opening in the duodenal wall. After we pass the opening, the walls are different and there isn't as much mucus. We'd better stop and figure out why there's such a big change in the landscape.

The first clue is that the pH meter has been getting quite a workout on this trip. Coming down through the stomach it registered a highly acid pH 2.0 and 2.5; we moved into the duodenum and it registered less acid at about 4.2; then we went by that hole in the duodenal wall and the needle bounced up to the alkaline 7 and 8 pH range. Whatever is coming out of that hole certainly has changed the pH readings.

We know that it's very acid in the stomach and that the chyme moves from the stomach into the duodenum. There are a lot of mucus-producing Brunner's glands in the duodenum to protect it from the acid. Yet as soon as we passed that opening, we noticed that there are fewer mucous glands. We must assume that additional protection isn't needed any more. It follows logically that the contents of this part of the small intestine should be less acid since the tissue of the walls isn't as well protected.

A quick check of our reference book tells us that the opening we passed is called the ampulla of Vater, or the papilla of Vater. This is where the common bile duct from the liver, gallbladder and pancreas empties into the duodenum. We had better see what's going on in there to cause the big change out here.

Slithering through the sphincter of Oddi that guards the opening at the ampulla of Vater puts us into the common bile duct. In here, as liquid cascades toward the opening, we get a deep appreciation of the plight of salmon swimming upstream. The amount of liquid coming down this duct totals about two quarts a day. A closer look tells us that it is pancreatic fluid and bile.

As we move along the common passageway, we come to a junction. The sign post tells us the right fork leads to the pancreas and the left to the gallbladder and liver. Since we're closer to the pancreas, we'll see what's going on in there first.

As we pass the fork in the duct and move into the pancreas, a quick check of the pH meter shows 8.0. A lot of clear fluid resembling saliva is coming out of the pancreas—enough to add up to nearly a quart a day.

When we reach the pancreas, we find it has two distinct but equally important functions. It produces both internal and external secretions. Although we can't see what's going on internally, hormones, including insulin, are being produced and delivered directly to the blood.

The external secretions are pancreatic juices; we can see these. There are three major enzymes in this juice, each with a specific role to help in the digestion process: protease for protein; lipase for digest fats; and carbohydrase for carbohydrates. Our reference books tell us that all of these enzymes work best in an alkaline environment—7.5 to 8.2 pH.[2] They also tell us that there is a lot of sodium bicarbonate secreted and that the pH of this sodium bicarbonate solution averages 8.0[3].

Now we can see why there was such a big change back there in the walls of the duodenum after we passed the ampulla of Vater. All of this alkaline pancreatic juice flows into the duodenum and neutralizes the chyme that comes from the stomach. You don't need Brunner's glands to produce tissue-protecting mucus when the contents of the intestine are alkaline.

We've solved the riddle of the changing landscape in the duodenum. As long as we're in the neighborhood, let's go up the other spur of the common bile duct.

Moving along the north fork headed toward the liver, we notice it isn't quite as pleasant here as it was in the pancreas. It is definitely more acid.

We come to an opening in this wall and, as soon as we pass it, the needle on the pH meter springs right back up to an alkaline reading. It appears we are now measuring the pH of bile as it comes directly from the liver.

Bile contains no enzymes, only substances that emulsify fats. Bile doesn't "digest" fats. It breaks them down so that they can be absorbed by the intestine and dealt with by other systems.

WELLNESS PRINCIPLE: *The liver always produces alkaline bile; if it can't do it the way it should, it won't do it at all.*

Everything coming out of the liver has a pH of 7.1 or above. It can be as high as 8.6. This is an exciting discovery, because it substantiates the claim that the body really knows what it is doing. Remember those pancreatic enzymes that work best in pH 7.5 to 8.2? This liver bile is going to be mixed with them in the common bile duct. Liver bile of 7.1 to 8.5 pH is going to be dumped in with 7.5 to 8.2 pH pancreatic juice that contains enzymes, and the liver bile pH won't interfere with enzymatic function at all.

Now that we've figured that out, we'll head back. But once again, as we come abreast of the opening labeled "gallbladder," our pH meter blips to a more acid reading. We'd better go in and take a look.

With meter in hand, we step inside the gallbladder. The meter needle plummets from pH 8.5 to 5.5. It looks as though we've stumbled onto another acid-producing organ. Yet our search of the reference books gives no hint that the gallbladder produces acid. They do tell us, however, that water and electrolytes (substances such as sodium, potassium, and chloride salts that conduct electric current)[4] are reabsorbed from the gallbladder. When these properties are taken out, the bile is concentrated and becomes thicker.

The gallbladder is the storage area for bile from the liver. Remember that the liver produces 7.1 to 8.5 pH bile. Yet this same bile, after it has been concentrated in the gallbladder, registers as low as pH 5.5. That's amazing! We must have missed something. There is no way to turn an alkaline substance into acid by concentrating it. If anything, taking only neutral substances away would make it an even more powerful alkali.

Let's look at what it takes to change an alkaline solution to an acid solution. You can do it in one of two ways. You can either add acid to it, or you can take the alkalizing substances from it.

We'd better sit down and think about this. We know that the body doesn't make mistakes. It certainly wouldn't have a 5.5 pH substance here in the gallbladder unless it is absolutely necessary. Everything else in this neighborhood is alkaline. Why would gallbladder bile be acid when (1) it is going to mix with alkaline pancreatic juice containing enzymes that need an alkaline environment, and (2) it is going to flow into the duodenum where acid stomach chyme needs to be neutralized?

It would appear that although acid gallbladder bile may be Normal, it certainly isn't Natural; so it must be Necessary.

Let's see what our reference books say about the physiological capabilities of the gallbladder. They tell us that the gallbladder can concentrate bile by removing sodium, bicarbonate, and chloride. These properties can be reabsorbed from the bile and put back into the bloodstream. Sodium can be removed from the gallbladder! That's interesting. I think we have found something *very* important. Gallbladder bile becomes acid when the alkaline properties are reabsorbed.

Perhaps the body isn't "making" acid gallbladder bile after all. Instead, the bile is "becoming" acid as a result of the body being forced to "rob Peter to pay Paul." Neutralizing elements are being "taken" from the gallbladder because they are urgently needed someplace else to take care of an even more crucial job. The gallbladder doesn't produce acid bile because it needs it as an end product; acid bile is a consequence of the body solving another problem someplace else. Looking at it this way, acid gallbladder bile is an effect, not a cause. Since the body never does anything without good reason, the alkaline properties taken from the gallbladder must be needed desperately for another function.

WELLNESS PRINCIPLE: *Sometimes it's easy to mistake the symptom for the problem.*

We had better take a closer look here inside the gallbladder to see what's going on. For one thing, there is a lot of thick sludge, rocks and boulders. Look at what we have been sitting on while reading our reference books and analyzing the situation—a gallstone! According to the books, gallstones in man are almost always made up of cholesterol and pigment[5], or a mixture of cholesterol, bilirubin, and protein[6].

Some of the conditions that bring about gallstones, our authorities tell us, are "too much" water, bile salts and lecithin being absorbed from the bile, and "too much" cholesterol being secreted into the bile. But this doesn't square with our perspective that the body doesn't do "too much" or "too little" of anything—everything the body does is correct. Nevertheless, stones aren't a part of the natural design, so there must be a good reason why they form.

Cholesterol constitutes the greatest portion of gallstones. Cholesterol is supposed to be in liquid form. It stays that way by its relationship to bile salts. However, in a gallbladder where stones form, the ratio of the cholesterol to bile salts has been upset. When the gallbladder takes sodium out of the bile, cholesterol is left to fend for itself. The cholesterol isn't a liquid any longer. It solidifies; and while we've been in here, we've been using it for a bench!

However, since we have said that the body never makes a mistake, why would it take sodium from the bile and leave solidifying cholesterol behind to cause all kinds of problems? There must be a very good reason.

Sodium is a primary contributor to the bicarbonate buffer system which is one of the systems that keeps the body from becoming too acid. If the person doesn't eat enough fruits and vegetables to provide organic sodium to work with the bicarbonate buffer system, the body will take the sodium from gallbladder bile. With the sodium gone, cholesterol is left high and dry to turn into stones. It is far more important for the body to be able to remain slightly alkaline than it is for it to prevent cholesterol from solidifying in the gallbladder. What difference does it make if stones are forming in the gallbladder if the alternative is for the body to become so acid that it can't function.

Your body will do everything it can to keep you alive—not necessarily to keep you comfortable and happy—just alive! It will attend to the most important things first in order to keep your cells functioning, and in this case it needs the sodium from the gallbladder to neutralize excess acid that is affecting your cells. We'll learn more about where the excess acid comes from after we complete our journey.

If sodium is taken from the gallbladder where it is serving an important, if not vital, function, we can assume that sodium is in short supply throughout the body. That explains why the saliva at the beginning of our journey was only 5.8 pH. There wasn't enough sodium in the body to keep the saliva alkaline. There is such a shortage of sodium that even when it is conscripted from the gallbladder, there's not enough to keep the saliva at its proper pH. Whatever process the sodium is being used for is much more crucial for sustaining life than are alkaline saliva and liquid gallbladder bile. If we had understood how this worked when we first entered the mouth, we would have realized that the 5.8 pH saliva reading was an indication that this body is in trouble.

This whole situation beautifully illustrates that everything that goes on in your body is in response to at least one stimulus and results in at least one effect.

WELLNESS PRINCIPLE: *No process of the body takes place in isolation.*

Solving the low-saliva pH and gallstone riddles also sheds light on why ulcers generally occur in the duodenum rather than in the stomach. Three-fourths of ulcers are duodenal ulcers. We can see from our vantage point inside the gallbladder that the alkaline bile originating in the liver becomes acid in the gallbladder before it gets to the common bile duct. The bile leaving the common bile duct should be alkaline so it can neutralize the acid chyme coming from the stomach. But if the alkaline liver bile and pancreatic juice have been contaminated with acid bile from the gallbladder, it can't neutralize acid chyme. Acid is being added to acid, and we know that strong acids can burn unprotected tissue. The walls of the duodenum are unprotected after the ampulla of Vater, so it becomes apparent that what we term a duodenal "ulcer" is really an acid bile burn!

WELLNESS PRINCIPLE: *Unprotected sensitive tissue that is designed to carry alkaline materials is defenseless against acid substances.*

Our observations of what is going on in the gallbladder are really exciting. We've seen things that reinforce our contention that the body never makes a mistake, and we've come to understand how some of the digestive problems that plague thousands of people are in reality the results of the body working intelligently to preserve itself.

We have so much food for thought, we had better abort our journey now and contemplate our observations.

We now know that gallbladder bile becomes acid only when sodium and other alkalizing elements are taken from it. We understand why bile leaving the common bile duct can be acid although it is supposed to be a neutralizing alkaline.

How can the problem of acid bile be resolved? There are two ways to return the alkalinity level of bile to normal. The best way is to change your diet so that there is plenty of organic sodium available throughout your body to meet the needs of the entire body. The other, far less desirable way is to remove the gallbladder so it can't pump acid bile into the system. This is about as effective as cutting off a foot to cure gout. The painful toe may be gone, but the condition that caused the symptoms runs rampant.

When we realize that everything the body does is to protect and/or sustain itself, we can see that removing a gallbladder to relieve pain is not going to solve the problem. The person will feel better, but only the symptoms have been relieved.

Friends or relatives who have had their gallbladders removed may bask in the comfort of their new gallbladder-free lives. They say they can eat anything they want without the pain they had before surgery. You can understand now why they feel better. You can also understand that they haven't really solved the underlying problem.

In reality, the problem has been compounded. The problem is that there isn't enough sodium to satisfy the body's requirements. When the gallbladder was intact, at least sodium was being reclaimed from liver bile. With the gallbladder gone, the sodium that would have been recycled is lost, thereby reducing the total sodium supply even more.

After the gallbladder is removed, the person may feel better, but his level of health has taken a serious turn for the worse.

Unless those who have had their gallbladder removed add enough alkalizing foods in the form of vegetables and fruits to their diets, their bodies are still in danger of becoming intolerably acidic. The problem hasn't gone away. The body still needs neutralizing minerals. Unless these minerals are supplied regularly by the diet, the body will find another source to carry on the function of the sodium that had previously been supplied by the gallbladder. Calcium is the most readily available substitute for sodium. The best source of calcium is the bones, and you know what happens when the bones lose more and more calcium—osteoporosis.

It would be interesting to see the results of a study of the incidence of osteoporosis in those who have had their gallbladders removed as compared with those who haven't.

WELLNESS PRINCIPLE: *With or without a gallbladder, everyone needs to eat fruits and vegetables to keep his supply of neutralizing minerals replenished.*

A few pages back, you may have begun to feel rather smug about your own sodium level if you eat the standard fare served in most homes and eating establishments around the country. In our society, we put salt on everything from breakfast eggs to margaritas. It seems almost impossible not to have enough sodium to handle the body's requirements. Unfortunately, table salt is different from the organically bonded sodium in fruits and vegetables. Our bodies don't use table salt. How do we know this? As we will see in Chapter 17, studies have shown that we eliminate as much sodium chloride each day as we take in. I am firmly convinced that ultimately investigations will confirm that inorganic table salt can't be easily broken apart by the body. Remember: *inorganic* = tightly held together; *organic* = easily broken apart. In a later chapter, I'll go into why the type of chemical bonds of minerals in our food is so important. For now, keep in mind that we can't beef up our sodium supply with salt on our steak.

The lessons we have learned on our excursion down the alimentary canal are crucial. They are paramount to understanding how the wrong types of food can cause major problems in unexpected areas. Let's recap.

1. Saliva should provide an environment where the enzyme ptyalin can work most effectively. The body doesn't put a substance in surroundings that inhibit its function unless it must in order to survive.

2. The stomach is the only place that needs acid solutions to function properly. It normally produces all of the acid necessary to prepare food for digestion.

3. Liquified food and digestive juices are emptied from the stomach into the duodenum. The resulting mixture, known as chyme, is acid.

4. The upper part of the duodenum can accept acidic substances from the stomach without being damaged, because Brunner's glands produce great quantities of protective mucus.

5. Mucus protection is not present in the duodenum after the opening to the common bile duct. Alkaline liver bile and pancreatic juices coming from the common bile duct neutralize the contents of the duodenum.

6. The liver produces about 1.75 pints of bile a day. About 95% is water. Bile includes cholesterol, bile pigments, bile salts, and

mineral salts. Production of liver bile is continuous. When bile is produced but not needed immediately, it is stored in the gallbladder.

7. The gallbladder can reclaim sodium, water and other elements from bile salts for use elsewhere in the body.

8. Bile becomes concentrated when water and bile salts are taken out.

9. Cholesterol loses its fluid nature when sodium is separated from the bile salts and is removed, along with other liquifying elements, from the bile.

10. Continuous concentration of gallbladder bile provides an opportunity for cholesterol to solidify. Cholesterol is the principal ingredient of most gallstones. Gallstones cause pain and can obstruct the opening of the gallbladder.

11. Gallbladder bile becomes more acid when alkaline properties are removed. Bile that should be alkaline becomes acid.

12. Acid gallbladder bile dumped into the common bile duct mixes with alkaline liver bile and pancreatic juice.

13. When gallbladder bile is acid, fluids from the common bile duct enter the duodenum in an acidic state rather than alkaline state. They add to the acid level of liquified food from the stomach instead of neutralizing it. The unprotected duodenum can then be burned by the acid chyme.

14. Acid bile burn in the duodenum masquerades as an "ulcer" and adds to the discomfort of indigestion and "heartburn."

15. The body must adapt its natural functions to handle large quantities of acid farther along the system.

16. Additional acid puts greater demands on the bicarbonate buffer system, calls for more sodium to be reclaimed by the gallbladder, and the cycle is perpetuated.

We'll go into more detail in the following chapters about other effects a shortage of organic sodium has on your body and what causes the shortage in the first place. This trip, however, illustrates the intertwining nature of all of the systems of your body. The key to providing enough of the proper minerals to keep your body from having to take essential elements from one job to do another is to eat the correct types of foods in correct proportions.

HEALTH HINT

Adding generous quantities of vegetables to your diet every day and fruits as often as possible will give you the sodium you need for natural physiological function.

The only sure-fire source of *appropriate* sodium to replenish the alkaline reserve is fruits and vegetables. In time, you can build up your alkaline reserve and your body can function more easily and efficiently. However, table salt just won't do the trick.

Your body *must* respond to everything you put in your mouth. Different kinds of foods cause different responses. Some leave an acid ash after they are digested; others leave an alkaline ash. The kind of ash that is left often has little to do with how acid the food itself is when you eat it. Oranges and lemons, for instance, are acid fruits, but they leave an alkaline ash. The secret to being healthy is to know which foods do what, and to keep a balance of the two kinds so that your body can function at its best.

HEALTH HINT

You DO NOT need to be a vegetarian to be healthy! And by the same token, being a vegetarian does not INSURE health. Ratios are the key factor. When you eat MORE vegetables and fruit than acid ash-producing foods, your body can maintain the necessary reserve of usable sodium. With adequate reserves, acid ash can be processed easily, other minerals are allowed to perform their functions, and good health follows.

By modifying your diet to provide more natural neutralizing minerals, all sorts of "symptoms" will disappear and you will be on your way to being genuinely healthy. The next chapter will explain how the ash residue of food dictates that your body adapt to necessary methods of physiological functioning.

CHAPTER 10

Reducing Your Food to Ashes

One of the last things you might expect to find in a book about health is a section on ashes. The ash we're talking about is not that left as remnants of a cheery log fire — but that's close. *Ash* is defined as an "incombustible powdery residue of a substance that has been completely incinerated."[1]

The ash we are talking about is the metabolic residue that is left after food has been digested and assimilated. During the digestive process, nutrients such as vitamins, minerals, enzymes, and other usable components of food are used or stored. Components of ash are either absorbed into the body or eliminated.

Ash is a residue of digested food that is different from the residue of bulk materials such as cellulose in celery, bran, and other foods that contain what we call roughage. Roughage is never really "taken into" the body. It passes through the intestinal tract without being assimilated and is eliminated through the bowel.

Both animal and vegetable foods leave an ash. The ash of animal protein, dairy products, eggs, and grains is generally acid. The ash of most fruits and vegetables is alkaline.

The difference between acid ash-producing foods and alkaline ash-producing foods is quite significant. Alkaline ash leaves alkalizing minerals the body can use to neutralize excess dietary acid. Alkaline ash is good! Our bodies are supposed to be slightly alkaline. Acid ash, on the other hand, leaves minerals that must be neutralized before

77

the body can dispose of them. Foods like meat, grains, and dairy products that are high in sulfur and phosphorus content have an acidifying effect.

The body is able to handle acidifying minerals in moderate quantities. However, if most of your food leaves acid ash, too much acid accumulates and the vital minerals of your alkaline reserve must be used to neutralize the acid. Your reserves will be emptied if the minerals are not replenished. If most of your food leaves acid ash (meat, grains, and dairy products), and only a small proportion leaves alkaline ash (vegetables and fruits), the acid level of your body will rise. This explains why it is so important that your diet be seventy-five percent fruits and vegetables and only twenty-five percent other foods.

Most foods grown in nature contain all of the elements you need for good nutrition. Yet, some foods have a higher percentage of acidifying minerals than others. When your diet is made up predominantly of acid ash-producing foods, excessive quantities of acid mineral residue are left to be dealt with. The residue contains strong acids such as sulfuric acid and phosphoric acid, that must be neutralized and eliminated by the kidneys. These strong acids cannot be exhaled as can carbonic acid from cellular metabolism and exercise.

Strong acids must be neutralized. Minerals of the alkaline reserve — sodium, calcium, potassium, and magnesium — perform the neutralizing function. If there is a little too much acid occasionally, the kidneys can take care of it. Too much acid on a regular basis is more than the kidneys can handle.

WELLNESS PRINCIPLE: *Too much acid ash leads to toxicity.*

A large percentage of our population lives on acid ash-producing foods. According to a report published in the *American Journal of Public Health*[2], on a typical day, forty percent of our population eats no fruit, and twenty percent allows no vegetables to pass their lips. In my opinion, these are overly conservative percentages; my personal estimate is more like eighty percent and forty percent. Is it any wonder that just about everyone you know complains of aches, pains, and illness?

If needed alkalizing minerals (from vegetables and fruits) aren't replaced, the body will adapt its natural functions to accommodate to conditions that are far from natural. It must adapt its functions and call on backup systems to handle what are, in essence, emergencies. In time, however, adaptation begins to take its toll. No system, or the body, can sustain "combat readiness" on a continuous basis without suffering from excess stress, and eventually breaking down. When this happens, we develop chronic degenerative diseases like osteoporosis, arthritis, multiple sclerosis, cancer, or AIDS. In the long term, our bodies process excess acid by using backup systems designed to get us through short-term crises.

Backup systems are ingenious devices designed to help your body tolerate excesses and abuses. However, expecting them to carry you through indefinitely is like depending on a temporary spare tire to do more than get you to the next filling station. Backup systems, like the spare, are designed to keep you going only until relief is available. When either is pushed beyond its limit, it will give out. The body can function on backup systems for only so long before symptoms of disease begin.

WELLNESS PRINCIPLE: *Backup systems, our safeguards against abuse, can be abused.*

Unfortunately, children are not immune to the ravages of the effects of too much acid ash food. Just because children haven't been around as many years as their parents doesn't mean they have an extended time-cushion before their natural health is in jeopardy. For one thing, they get a head start on toxicity if their mothers followed an acidifying diet during pregnancy. Before they are born, children are subjected to the rewards or penalties of the diets and lifestyles of their mothers.

Consequently, it isn't unusual these days to see twenty-year olds with physiological problems that once were seen almost exclusively in sixty-year olds. This is understandable when you consider relatively recent innovations in food processing. Refined foods, fast-foods, and high-tech processed foods are quite new on the scene. Other relatively modern "advancements" are refined white flour and white sugar, hormone-fed livestock, hybrid and mutated produce, and synthetic "foods" such as "non-dairy" milk, cream, and cheese, and "cholesterol-free egg" products. Food isn't what it was only a few generations ago. Sophisticated food processing, along with the addition of chemical preservatives other than salt, has come into its own in about the past twenty years.

One of the most recent wrinkles on the food treatment scene is irradiation. Selected foods are bombarded with gamma rays from radioactive isotopes as a method of killing insects, slowing ripening, or dehydration. Irradiation lengthens the unrefrigerated shelf-life of foods and slows the maturing process of fruits and vegetables so that they at least "look better" longer. Currently in the U.S., only a limited variety of food, including fresh pork, may legally be irradiated. Since irradiation brings about "formation of electrically charged highly reactive molecules that damage living cells,"[3] only time will determine the effects this high-technology procedure will have on the health of those who eat irradiated food.

All adults have been exposed to highly processed, adulterated food for about the same length of time. This is why in my clinic we see twenty- and forty-year olds with symptoms that used to show up mainly in people sixty years old, or older.

WELLNESS PRINCIPLE: *Toxicity from food has a cumulative effect.*

You may have heard people say things like, "I don't know what happened to me. After I turned forty, my health just broke. I wasn't sick a day until then, and I've been sick every day since." What happened is that the body had enough stored mineral reserves to hold up for forty years. The person was in trouble twenty years before, but his body still fought and fought until the reserves ran out when he hit age forty.

Along with the advances of technology has come a generally higher standard of living. This includes not only centrally heated and air-conditioned houses and work places, multiple-bathroom homes, VCRs, and photosensitive night lights, but also more meat in the average American's daily diet. The old political cliche "a chicken in every pot" was a tempting promise in the lean years of the depression. Meat, including chicken, was a treat for many. It wasn't the daily star of the show complemented by vegetables, beans, and grains. Carbohydrates and starches played the major roles in diets a scant 60 to 100 years ago.

However, these days, eating meat isn't the problem. Eating *too much* meat and other high-protein, acid ash-producing food is the problem! And not eating fruits and vegetables in sufficient proportions to replace the neutralizing materials of your alkaline reserve compounds the problem. Your body must deal with excessive amounts of acid metabolic residue, but the supplies it needs aren't replaced.

WELLNESS PRINCIPLE: *Continuous large amounts of animal protein leave more acid ash than the body can handle healthfully.*

Metabolic ash may not look like the dry, powdery residue you douse before you leave a campfire site, but it has many of the same properties.

When wood is burned, energy is produced. Food is the fuel for the body that is oxidized to produce energy. Food produces internal energy to maintain a constant temperature and to keep your organs and systems functioning. Both wood that is burned (oxidized) and food that is oxidized (burned) leave an ash. The alkalinity or acidity of the ash depends upon the composition of the substance burned.

For example, wood, with all of its elements intact before burning, is neither acid nor alkaline. It registers a neutral 7.0 pH. When neutral wood burns, the smoke coming from it is acid (smoke contains carbon dioxide). If you were to add a couple of drops of distilled water to the ash of burned wood and test it with pH paper, you would get an alkaline reading.

You can do the same thing to food to determine whether the residual ash is acid or alkaline. If you perform a home chemistry experiment to test the pH of an orange, you will find that the meat of orange sections fresh out of their skin is quite acidic. Oranges contain a lot of citric acid. You can take a couple of sections of that orange, put them into a stainless steel container, and "ash" them in a self-cleaning oven. The orange slices will oxidize, leaving only a white powder. The extreme heat converts cellulose and other materials that make up the whole fruit into carbon dioxide and other gasses. If you moisten the residual powdery ash with a few drops of distilled water and test the pH, the ash will register alkaline. This demonstra-

tion illustrates that there can be a marked difference between the pH
of the original food and the pH of the ash of that food.

Essentially, the same basic process of oxidation that went on in
the oven takes place in your body. Food is taken in, broken down to
cell-size portions, and "burned." Of course, the process isn't nearly as
hot or as fast as it is in an oven or open fire. The body is quite sedate
in "burning" foods. It works more slowly than direct heat sources,
and it works at much lower temperatures. Yet the end result is the
same. The ash that is left is a mineral residue that won't burn.

There is a mineral residue left from the oxidation of most of the
food you eat. Many foods that are obviously acidic, such as oranges,
grapefruit, and apricots, leave an alkaline ash. On the other hand,
foods that seem to be quite benign, like soda crackers and chicken
soup, can leave an acid ash or have an acidifying effect on the body.
It is the minerals in the residue that are acid or alkaline, not the food
itself. Understanding the difference between foods that are acid in
their original form and foods that are acid-producing can be very important to your health.

WELLNESS PRINCIPLE: *The ash of food is rarely of the same
pH as that of the food in the form
that you ate it.*

Some foods leave no ash but have an acidifying effect on the
body. Although the food doesn't leave an ash, the food is metabolized by the cells. All cells produce acid as they function, consequently, acid is produced by the cells as the foods are processed.
Syrups, fats, oils, white sugar, and some other processed or synthetic
foods fall into the "no ash" category. You get a great surge of energy
after eating them because the body works very hard and fast to metabolize them. All of this activity produces a lot of energy, but it also
produces a lot of acid. This is why we say some foods, such as white
sugar, leave no ash but have an acidifying effect.

To illustrate how this works, you can ash sugar beets in your
oven. Carbon dioxide (which is acid) will burn off and the ash that is
left will be alkaline. However, if sugar beets are refined into white
sugar and then the white sugar is ashed, the carbon dioxide will be
burned off but there will be no residue—no ash.

In the same way, when you eat white sugar, there's no ash left. A lot of energy is produced, however, and the carbon dioxide from the oxidation process is exhaled. Seems harmless enough. The bad news is that the acid produced by the activity of the cells adds to the overall acid level, yet the sugar doesn't contribute any beneficial minerals. Proportions are upset. The acid level is increased but no new neutralizing minerals are supplied to neutralize the strong acids from other foods that can't be eliminated through the lungs. This may provide a clue to the close association between sugary foods and the hyperactivity of some children. Their overly acid bodies are showing telltale signs of hyper-irritability common to acidosis. It would appear that we are all affected by sugar, but some of us have more intense responses than others.

WELLNESS PRINCIPLE: *White sugar is too potent a food for us – it stimulates physiological activity but doesn't replace the enzymes, vitamins, or minerals needed to process it.*

By contrast, look at what happens when you eat a carrot. The carrot is broken down and the constituent elements are absorbed into the bloodstream. Some of the cellulose of the carrot is not digested. Cellulose is residue that never really gets "into" the body. Residue goes directly to the intestine to be eliminated in the feces. None of the cellulose of the carrot was involved in the metabolic process. In essence, it never really "entered" the body. Cellulose provides no nutritional benefits, although it does provide fiber that is helpful for the bowels and elimination.

The food we eat (including the carrot) contains many different substances, and all food provides glucose for the cells to use.

Once the usable parts of the carrot are digested, glucose and the other nutrients are absorbed into the bloodstream. We get energy from glucose. The body tears apart the organic bonds that hold together the elements of glucose—carbon, hydrogen, and oxygen. This activity produces acid inside the cell in the same way as breaking apart the bonds of glucose of white sugar. But here's the big difference. The mineral residue of the carrot has an alkalizing effect on the body. Alkaline minerals such as sodium, potassium, calcium, and magnesium are left to neutralize accumulated physiological acids. The neutralizers can be used immediately if necessary; or they can be stored as a part of the alkaline reserve for future neutralizing jobs. Carrots haven't cornered the alkaline mineral market; most vegetables and fruits leave a life-enriching legacy of alkaline minerals.

WELLNESS PRINCIPLE: *Alkaline ash foods replenish your alkaline reserve.*

When parts of food are assimilated into the body, that food works either for us or against us. Going through the digestive tract is rather like going through a tunnel. Until the bits and pieces are absorbed into the many systems of the body to be worked on and turned into energy, they are inside the tunnel, but not really contributing anything.

To use another analogy, gasoline in your car's gas tank, fuel lines, and pumps doesn't fire the engine. The fuel must get to the energy-producing mechanisms before it can act for good or mischief. It doesn't make any difference whether you put high octane unleaded gas or diesel fuel in a fuel tank until you try to operate the engine. That's when the quality of fuel becomes known.

Food works in the same way. The big difference is that once food goes in, the body will work with it. You can't turn off your digestive system and put your body up on blocks. That being the case, you're better off making sure you have the right fuel — at least most of the time — to keep your physiological engine running smoothly.

The jumping-off place for food assimilation in the body is the small intestine. This is where most of the elements of the foods you have eaten are absorbed into the body so that the cells can work with them. Through the body's "selective service" capabilities, cells perform specialized functions. However, in order to do anything, cells need energy. When the energy-bearing food particles include acid ash, the cells must handle this also, and cell efficiency is reduced.

Remember, we live or die at the cellular level. When your cells are in trouble, you are in trouble. The problem with eating mostly acid ash foods is that your *cells* have to deal with the acid that's produced. They can get bogged down in acid. Then the intracellular pH, that should always be around 6.8, falls. When the pH is too low, enzymes can't work and other life- and health-sustaining processes assigned to that cell can't take place naturally.

Your life isn't going to be changed radically if twenty or thirty of your 75 trillion cells are abused. But if a high percentage is involved and can't function according to the original design of your internal intelligence, you can be assured that unpleasant symptoms will become evident. Your body's natural operational equilibrium will become unbalanced; your resistance will plummet; and disease will move in and take over.

The following lists show some common foods according to the type of ash they leave.

ALKALINE ASH AND ACID ASH FOODS[4,5]
ALKALINE ASH FOODS

Almonds	Dates, dried	Peaches
Apples	Figs, dried	Pears
Apricots	Grapefruit	Pineapple
Avocados	Grapes	Potatoes, sweet
Bananas	Green beans	Potatoes, white
Beans, dried	Green peas	Radishes
Beet greens	Lemons	Raisins
Beets	Lettuce	Raspberries
Blackberries	Lima beans, dried	Rhubarb**
Broccoli	Lima beans, green	Rutabagas
Brussels sprouts	Limes	Sauerkraut
Cabbage	Milk, goat's*	Soy beans, green
Carrots	Millet	Spinach, raw
Cauliflower	Molasses	Strawberries
Celery	Mushrooms	Tangerines
Chard leaves	Muskmelon	Tomatoes
Cherries, sour	Onions	Watercress
Cucumbers	Oranges	Watermelon
	Parsnips	

*Recommended only for infants for whom mother's milk is not available. See section on Goat's Milk, page 87.
**Not recommended–Rhubarb leaves an alkaline ash; however, it has other properties that are detrimental to the body

NEUTRAL ASH FOODS THAT HAVE

AN ACIDIFYING EFFECT

Corn oil   Refined sugar
Corn syrup   Olive oil

ACID ASH FOODS

Bacon	Currants	Pork
Barley	Eggs	Prunes~
Beef	Flour, white	Rice, brown
Blueberries	Flour, whole wheat	Rice, white
Bran, wheat	Haddock	Salmon
Bran, oat	Honey	Sardines
Bread, white	Lamb	Sausage
Bread, whole wheat	Lentils, dried	Scallops
Butter	Lobster	Shrimp
Carob	Milk, cow's ~	Spaghetti
Cheese	Macaroni	Squash, winter
Chicken	Oatmeal	Sunflower seeds
Codfish	Oysters	Turkey
Corn	Peanut butter	Veal
Corned beef	Peanuts	Walnuts
Crackers, soda	Peas, dried	Wheat germ
Cranberries~	Pike	Yogurt
	Plums~	

~These foods leave an alkaline ash but have an acidifying effect on the body

The concept that foods have acid-producing and alkaline-producing qualities is not brand new. Dr. R. A. Richardson listed foods by these categories in 1925.[6]

You probably noticed that the alkaline ash foods are essentially fruits and vegetables and that acid ash foods are generally meats-poultry-fish, dairy products, and grains. If we continue to follow the traditionally recommended pattern, we can be reasonably sure that we are going to end up with a real health problem. Our bodies are three-fourths alkaline, yet we are told to replenish and refuel them with three-fourths acid-producing foods.

GOAT'S MILK

Goat's milk appears in the alkaline ash list and cow's milk appears in the acid ash list. The subject of milk in general is covered in Chapter 18, "Osteoporosis by the Quart."

Human mother's milk is the ideal food for infants until after the child has acquired a few teeth. Unfortunately, some mothers are unable to nurse their babies. For those newborns and infants who must be fed something other than mother's milk, the closest acceptable substitute is a combination of fresh raw goat's milk, fresh carrot juice, and distilled water. For a newborn, the goat's milk, carrot juice, and distilled water are combined in equal thirds. As the child gets older, the amount of water is gradually decreased as the milk and carrot juice are increased. When the child is approximately six months old, the proportions should be fifty percent goat's milk and fifty percent carrot juice.

Cow's milk should be avoided. Cow's milk is fine for calves, but not for humans, either adults or children.

As a nation, we need to realize that the way we are eating is undermining our most precious resource — our health. Only by modifying our diets to provide the materials our bodies need to function naturally can we reverse the trend of serious disease proliferation. The effort required to modify eating habits is insignificant when weighed against the penalty for continuing health-ravaging diets. Merely by adding more alkaline ash producing foods to our daily meals, we can live more comfortable, satisfying lives.

However, a word of caution:

HEALTH HINT

Changing your diet to a more healthful balance of acid ash and alkaline ash foods should be done slowly. *Quick, radical changes may lead to long-term health but short-term misery.*

I have had patients suddenly develop "nutrition religion" and take one giant leap off of their standard high-protein diets into a regimen of raw fruits and vegetables. Invariably, within a few days, they painfully take refuge in their old ways. If you are now eating the current standard American high-protein diet, your body has adapted to accommodate those foods. Your metabolic activity doesn't change overnight. You need to gradually introduce more cooked vegetables and fruit into your system to let it slowly work back into functioning naturally. Otherwise, you will feel terrible and become convinced that all of this "eat better–feel better" hype is a bunch of balderdash.

WELLNESS PRINCIPLE: *Improve your diet like a shot, and you'll be more healthy but think you're not.*

So before you make any drastic dietary changes, let your body have a chance to get used to dealing with more wholesome food that includes the nutrients it was designed to handle but hasn't had in a long time. When your body is exposed to unusual circumstances, you feel repercussions. Changing your diet is similar to changing your physical activity level. Shoveling snow or putting in a garden will elicit temporary "pain and suffering" if your muscles have been on an extended vacation. Even though they were designed to do what you are asking of them, if they are not accustomed to vigorous activity, there will be a period of discomfort. Other systems of your body respond in much the same way. Asking your digestive and assimilative systems to make rapid radical changes throws them off balance for a short period also.

When you decide to improve your diet, give your digestive system the same consideration you give your muscles when you undertake a new exercise program. As with other "physical conditioning" programs, you need to start out slowly. Before you begin revamping your eating habits, you should have an idea of how healthy you are. When you know where you are right now, it's a whole lot easier to know how far you have to go.

CHAPTER 11

How to Check Your Level of Health

High cholesterol, low blood sugar, high blood pressure, electrolyte imbalance, weak eyes, shallow respiration, ruptured disc, or flat feet— there is a "test" to determine if you have fallen victim to one of these "abnormalities." But do diagnostic tests really give a true picture of how healthy you are, or do they merely point out particular problem areas?

In general, we equate "being healthy" with being symptom-free. For most of us, if we feel reasonably good, have a fair amount of energy, and our moving parts are in moderately good working order, we consider ourselves "healthy." However, there is more to health than not hurting.

"Health" in our society is calculated in terms of the *disease model*. For example, we operate on the premise that the body is a chemical factory and that a person gets sick if the chemicals are out of balance. To balance the chemicals, add a pinch of this and a speck of that and the person will get well. Simple as all that.

Unfortunately, the true health of your internal environment is not always revealed by your outward appearance or how you feel. Furthermore, lab tests at your annual physical can't do much to forecast future ailments. An accurate interpretation of the tests may predict that you are in a "high risk" category for a particular affliction. Essentially, though, lab tests are designed to find out if a particular condition has already progressed to the problem, or

89

pathologic, stage. What we need is a way to get an accurate picture of how healthy we are before symptoms appear. The good news is that just such a method is available.

Now you can draw your own picture of your health easily and inexpensively. All you need is a roll of pH test paper, a record chart, and a pencil. The substance you will monitor is readily available though not often discussed in polite society—urine. Simple tests of this waste material can give vital information about how healthy you are today and what you can expect in the future if your body continues to function as it is right now.

> **WELLNESS PRINCIPLE:** *Urine pH levels are highway signs on the road to health.*

Urine pH indicates the environmental conditions in which cells live and function. Remember, we live or die at the cellular level.

Your body's vast network of systems works best when the pH of fluids hovers around neutral to slightly alkaline. Urine pH can tell you if your body is holding its alkaline advantage or if it has slipped too far to the acid side.

Urine pH shows how your body handled the food you ate within the past 24 hours. It indicates how well your body is functioning.

Monitoring the pH of urine gives vital clues to what is going on in the body and how drastically it is adapting its functions. Remember, the body never makes a mistake! It always responds perfectly to every stimulus it receives. This is why it is so important that you understand the messages urine pH is sending you.

Keep in mind that the only things your body has to work with to replenish and rebuild cells are the elements and compounds that make up the food you eat.

The food you ate yesterday was broken down, parts of it were assimilated, used or stored, and other parts were discarded. The first urine of the morning contains much of the material that has been processed-out while you were sleeping. While you sleep, your body is busy repairing, restoring, and replenishing cells, tissue, and organs. At the same time, it prepares unusable residue, toxins, and other extraneous parts of food for elimination.

If you have a lot of debris to be discarded, your sleep may be interrupted for a trip to the bathroom. The urine you eliminate after four or five hours of sleep contains the junk your body doesn't need and can't use. Urine is a vehicle for removing substances from the body.

WELLNESS PRINCIPLE: *The first urine pH of the morning tells how your body handled the food you ate yesterday.*

Testing your body's pH is quite simple and inexpensive. You will need pH paper test strips calibrated in two-tenths increments to get a reasonably accurate reading. Paper that registers between pH 5.5 and 8.0 is suitable for most people. Some pH paper shows differences in full units—4.0, 5.0, 6.0 and so forth—but these readings are not accurate enough for our purposes.

Recall that there is a tenfold change in intensity between each pH unit. For example, when a reading drops (from pH 6 to pH 5, for example), this indicates that the acidity of the solution increases. The numbers go up as solutions become less acid. The degree of alkalinity leaps by ten times from one whole number to the next.

Because there is such a vast change between two units and the changes that take place in pH readings can be extremely slight from one week to the next, you need test paper that is highly sensitive in order for some small but significant variations to register. If you use test strips calibrated in full units, it may take several months for changes brought about by diet to become evident. This is why it's important to use test paper calibrated in two-tenths increments. You may be able to get this kind of paper from your pharmacist or local surgical supply firm. If it is not available from either of those sources, you can write to the address at the front of this book.

Once you have acquired pH paper that registers in appropriate increments, you are ready to begin keeping a record of your fluid readings using the charts found at the end of this chapter. Casually checking your pH readings during the day doesn't tell you much. In order to gain insight into your health, you need a little organization in your research. You can do this by following a simple, flexible schedule. However, it is important to stick to the designated types of food in order to get an accurate picture.

WELLNESS PRINCIPLE: *The kind of food you eat dictates how your body responds.*

Instructions for monitoring your health appear to be much more involved than the procedure really is. Actually, all you need to do is dip pH paper into the fluid you are testing, compare the color of the wet pH strip, and record the results. The instructions that follow are more detailed and explain why you do the test at particular times.

TESTING URINE pH

The first order of business when you get up in the morning is to catch some urine in a small, clean container. Test the pH of the fluid with the pH test paper. When the paper is wet, the change in color should be obvious. If it isn't obvious, you may need pH paper designed to register at a lower pH range.

Compare the color of the paper with the colors shown on the gauge that comes with the paper, and record the pH number on the Health Profile Monitoring Chart found at the end of this chapter. Ideally, you should check your urine pH after you have slept nonstop for at least five hours and your body has had a chance to do some internal house cleaning.

If your sleep is interrupted, take the reading after the longest period of uninterrupted sleep, even if it's three o'clock in the morning. Also record how long you slept. Over time, as your health improves and your pH numbers get better, you will find that you are sleeping more soundly for longer periods. Of course, if children are waking you during the night, your diet won't have much effect on their sleeping habits—but their diets will. Children really benefit from improved eating habits!

WELLNESS PRINCIPLE: *Get healthy for the rest of your life.*

To establish your pH baseline, check your urine pH first thing in the morning after you have eaten the foods you customarily eat the night before.

That's all there is to checking urine pH—once in the morning, and the first time establishes your baseline.

WHAT TO EAT WHILE MONITORING pH

In order to get a clear picture of your level of health after you have established your baseline, eat only acid ash foods for two days. (Refer to pages 85-86 for appropriate menu items.) The purpose of dumping acid ash foods into your system is to set up a temporary "worst case scenario" for your body to handle in order to get the most reliable research results.

The "worst case" for your body is to deny it any of the materials it needs to process and dispose of the acid generated by an excessive amount of protein. For two days, you contrive to give your body only a heavy load of protein. Foods such as steak, or its less grand protein-rich cousins, hamburger, chicken, fish, or macaroni and cheese leave acid ash.

You may have noticed that you are rather thirsty when you eat high-protein meals. During the monitoring period, drink only water. If you must have coffee, tea, or soft drinks, limit your consumption to two cups or less each day.

Although you don't want to inflict high-protein abuse on your body frequently, it can tolerate it for a couple of days. The extreme conditions provide the best setting to determine how your overall health is holding up.

RECAP OF THREE-DAY MONITORING

Day One: (1) Begin monitoring urine pH with the first voiding in the morning after a day when you have eaten the foods you usually eat. The numbers you get for Day One will serve as a baseline.

(2) Eat only acid ash-producing foods (meats, dairy, grains, nuts, etc.). You may need to plan ahead for these meals if you ordinarily eat generous quantities of vegetables.

(3) Drink only water, if possible. If not, limit coffee, tea, cola or other beverages to two cups or less each day. Avoid alcoholic drinks and fruit juices.

Day Two: A repeat of Day One. Only acid ash-producing foods and water or limited quantities of other drinks.

Day Three: You can revert to your usual diet after you take a
                    reading based on Day Two's food.

HOW HEALTHY CAN YOU
EXPECT TO BECOME?

Monitoring your urine pH tells you how your body is handling
the food you eat from day to day. There is another quick test you can
perform with pH paper that is an indicator of how well your body is
functioning as a whole—the saliva test. Saliva is representative of all of
the internal fluids of your body. When your internal environment is
alkaline, your saliva is alkaline.

You may want to establish a baseline for your saliva pH at about
the same time you establish the baseline for urine pH. You don't
have to check your saliva pH every day; it changes very slowly. Every
two or three weeks after you have started to improve your diet, check
your saliva pH and record the results. By keeping a record, you will
be able to see quantitative evidence of how the climate of your internal environment is progressing.

To check saliva pH, put some saliva into a spoon, dip the pH test
paper into it, and compare the color of the paper with the color
gauge on the dispenser.

> **CAUTION:** *A few people are so sick that they are
> highly sensitive or allergic to the chemicals in the test
> paper. For this reason, it is advisable for you not to
> put the chemically treated paper in your mouth.*

The purpose of testing saliva is to compare pH readings before
and after eating a meal. Check your saliva pH before you eat, then
again about four minutes after you eat. Record the results for comparisons in the future.

If you prefer, there is another way to check your saliva pH without having to wait for mealtime. The lemon test provides the physiological stimulus of a "mini-meal." It brings about a physiological
reaction that can be monitored with pH paper.

Sometime during the day after you have had nothing to eat for two hours, check your saliva pH and write down the results. Then take the Lemon Test. All you need is a fresh lemon and pH paper.

LEMON TEST

Check your saliva pH after having had nothing to eat for two hours or more. Take this reading before you even pick up the lemon. For some people, just handling the little rascal has been known to send the saliva pH soaring.

Squeeze a teaspoonful of juice into a spoon or glass of water and drink it (it is perfectly acceptable to shudder and grimace). Wait two minutes, then check your saliva pH again.

The highly acid lemon juice creates a high stress condition for your body that calls for maximum saliva production. The normal alkalinity of your mouth is disrupted by the acid in the lemon juice. Salivary amylase, or ptyalin, a major enzyme found in saliva, is an enzyme that is effective only in an alkaline environment. Lemon juice quickly changes the environment of your mouth to intense acidity. To counteract this, your body goes to work immediately to return the pH to normal by flooding the mouth with neutralizing saliva. With the initial flooding, saliva pH usually shoots up to its highest readings, then gradually drops back to its normal level.

WHAT DO THE NUMBERS MEAN?

If you have followed the game plan, you are ready to evaluate your level of health based on information of more substance than merely "feeling good" or "feeling bad." For the first time, you have reliable information on your own personal Health Index. Of course, data are only as good as their interpretation. In the next chapter, we'll look at what the numbers mean to your present and future health.

HEALTH PROFILE
MONITORING CHART

# Hours Of Sleep	Monitoring	Urine pH
	Day One Baseline Eat Acid Ash-Producing Food	
	Day Two Eat Acid Ash-Producing Food	
	Day Three Eat Regular Food	

CHAPTER 12

Interpreting Your Data

Several years ago, I had a young patient with whom I had discussed nutrition only briefly. He was a strapping young man, a former Green Beret intently interested in health and fitness. We had talked about the negative effects of acid on the body and how the kind of food you eat can dramatically increase acid levels. I had given him some pH paper and instructed him on the types of foods he should eat while monitoring his pH.

He went away to confirm what he knew to be his superior level of health. A few days later he came back into the office and announced triumphantly, "See, I told you, Doc, vegetables are bad for you." I found this a rather startling statement and pressed for an explanation.

He pulled out his monitoring chart to show me that when he ate roast beef, Parkerhouse rolls, and brown rice, his urine pH registered a healthful 7.4. But after he had eaten nothing but fruits and vegetables for a day or two, his urine pH plummeted to 5.5—off the chart. He was delighted to have "disproved" my contention that the body needs fruits and vegetables to maintain its natural alkaline nature.

What he had not realized was that his readings staunchly reinforced my concept. His readings were a classic demonstration that confirmed all I had been telling him. His pH was high after a day of acid ash foods and protein, and low after a day of vegetables and

97

fruit. This pattern indicated that his alkaline reserve was perilously low.

In the chapters that follow, you will learn why he got the readings he did, why you get the readings you do, and how you can adjust your patterns for living to help you improve not only your numbers but, more important, your health!

> **WELLNESS PRINCIPLE:** *pH readings are indicators of health.*

This chapter will give you the "key" for scoring your level of health according to your urine pH readings. Your "score" will give you the most accurate gauge of how much your body is adapting its Natural functions to those that are Necessary to keep it going. Even if you are completely free of symptoms, your body may be working in ways that assure eventual disease.

The concepts behind the interpretations of your pH will be explained in the succeeding chapters. For now, it is important for you to keep in mind that the body *must* have a particular kind of sodium (organic) in order to be able to neutralize acid. When organic sodium is present in adequate amounts, urine pH registers as an acid after you have eaten acid ash foods. If you don't have enough reserve sodium, your urine pH will register alkaline after you eat predominantly acid ash foods. This may sound topsy-turvy to you now, but the reasoning will soon become more clear to you. But, first things first:

WHAT YOUR URINE pH READINGS MEAN

With numbers as a guide, you can evaluate how well your body is functioning. If your Health Index scores indicate your body is responding appropriately to the food you eat, congratulations. You are among a fortunate minority. If your scores indicate that you are headed for trouble and you choose to continue to do the things you have been doing, you shouldn't be surprised when you begin to feel less and less well and to experience more and more symptoms of disease. The choice is yours. First, the key for scoring urine pH and for determining your own Health Index following the three-day monitoring period:

HEALTH INDEX SCORECARD
According to your urine pH

Third Day Urine pH	After a Controlled Diet of ACID ASH FOODS (*Meats, Dairy, Grains, etc.*)
6.8 - 8.0	POSSIBLE DISASTER PENDING
6.0 - 6.6	AT RISK
5.5 - 5.8	MINERAL RESERVES AVAILABLE*

*NOTE "Mineral Reserves Available" means just that: It doesn't guarantee the condition will be maintained unless the minerals that are being lost are replaced.

Keep in mind that urine pH tells you how your body handled the food you ate the day before. The 5.5 to 5.8 pH category shows the most favorable physiological response to acid ash foods. However, as you will see, it is precisely this response, day after day, year after year, that ultimately causes the physiological mayhem that leads to disease.

Those whose third-day readings register in the ranges of 6.0 to 6.6, or 6.8 to 8.0, at some time in the past had readings that registered 5.5 to 5.8. They didn't start out in the "At Risk" or "Disaster Pending" groups. They used up their mineral supplies by eating too many acid ash foods and they neglected to replenish their supplies with minerals from alkaline ash foods. Over time, their pH numbers have gone up and up. We will see later that alkaline urine following an acid ash meal is the result of the body adapting to protect itself.

If your reserves of neutralizing minerals are adequate, when you eat acid ash producing foods, your urine pH will register an acidic 5.8 or lower the next morning. Although this may appear to be backwards, it is the ideal response of a well-stocked alkaline reserve.

Why is your urine slightly acid if your alkaline reserve is in great shape? Why isn't the urine alkaline with all of those helpful neutralizing minerals available? The answer to these questions lies in understanding why and how urine becomes alkaline or acid.

The acid residue of meat and other acid ash-producing foods is strong and dangerous to the urinary tract. Strong acids must be neutralized or weakened. Acid urine is neutralized in one of two ways: either alkaline minerals are added, or, if appropriate minerals are not available, ammonia is used. Ammonia as a urine neutralizer is an emergency backup system. Ammonia is more highly alkaline than alkaline reserve minerals. It has a pH of about 9.25.

So we have a strong acid that is going to be eliminated in the urine and two methods of neutralizing it: (1) the alkaline reserve, if any, and (2) the emergency backup, ammonia.

When moderately alkaline minerals are taken from the alkaline reserve and added to the strong acid, the strong acid is made weaker.

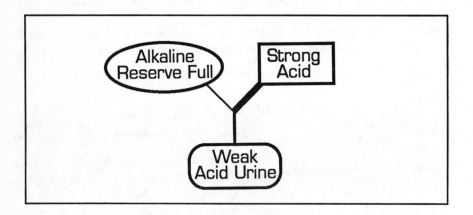

It is still acid, but weak enough not to irritate delicate tissue.

If the alkaline reserve has been depleted, minerals aren't available from that source to buffer the acid. Yet the body is intent upon survival. It will neutralize the strong acid even if it has to alter its normal way of functioning. One of the alterations it makes is to use ammonia produced by the body. Ammonia is used to neutralize the strong acid. Again, ammonia is a very strong alkali. It overpowers the acid and the urine registers highly alkaline, around pH 8.0 or higher.

The only reason the urine is alkaline when acid ash foods are being processed is because the body has adapted its function to take care of a dangerous situation. Alkaline urine following a meal of acid producing food is a sure sign that the alkaline reserve is depleted and that the body's resistance is faltering.

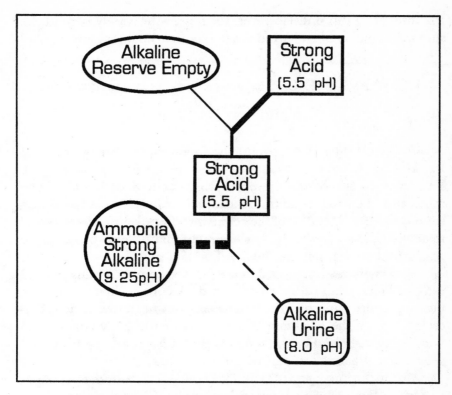

The neutralizing, or buffering, processes of the body will be described in greater detail in later chapters. Once you grasp the concept that alkaline urine following an acid meal is a sign of impending disaster, you will be better aware of what the food you eat is doing to or for your body.

WELLNESS PRINCIPLE: *Slight alkalinity is ideal, but weak acid is better than strong acid.*

If your readings show that you still have alkalizing minerals available, your alkaline reserve is holding its own. Right now, you are healthy. Currently, you have enough sodium to handle the harmful effects of eating excessive amounts of acid-ash producing foods. This doesn't mean you should eat them all of the time; it just means you can still handle them. If you eat excessive amounts of protein and other acid ash-producing foods, your supply of buffering materials will ultimately run out. However, for now, your supply is good. Be sure to eat plenty of fruits and vegetables to keep it that way.

   WELLNESS PRINCIPLE: *Your body works to maintain slight*
   alkalinity.

If after eating acid ash producing foods your morning urine pH was between 6.8 and 8.0, you are sick no matter how good you feel. You have already passed the point where your body has alkalizing minerals to be used to neutralize acid ash. Your body has lost the resources needed to get rid of the acidifying effects of food in a normal manner. Consequently, the backup ammonia system comes to the rescue and urine is neutralized for elimination.

Those who eat few acid ash foods (and remember, grains are acid ash producers) and whose customary diets consist chiefly of vegetables and fruits will ordinarily have alkaline urine. It makes no difference whether the alkalinity is the result of the body adapting to handle acid ash food or the result of the body processing fruits and vegetables. Alkaline urine turns pH paper dark.

Alkaline urine from fruits and vegetables can turn the pH paper as dark as alkaline urine laced with ammonia. The first is very good. The second is very bad.

It is good when the paper turns dark to indicate alkaline urine as a result of eating a high concentration of alkaline ash-producing foods. It's bad when it turns dark because you've eaten a steak and your urine pH is 7.0. Your body didn't have enough sodium to get rid of the acid from the steak in an acid form, so the body switched to a backup system and made an alkaline urine out of it. Urine that is alkaline because the backup system kicked in has an ammonia odor.

The odor of ammonia is considered by many to be normal for urine; however, it is a telltale sign that the body is using an emergency systems to keep going. *Most* Americans have been eating predominantly acid ash foods for most of their lives. They have already gone through their reserve of minerals, and their bodies have adapted to make up for the deficiency. Sometimes, it doesn't take years for this to happen. All too often, the ammonia odor of babies' diapers confirm that children can be victims of diet-induced mineral deprivation. Unfortunately, the results can be tragic.

HEALTH HINT

If your pH picture shows an alkaline urine after eating acid ash foods, begin today to replenish your alkaline reserve. Include one serving of raw fruit and cooked vegetables in your daily menus.

If your urine pH is high, as you add mineral-rich foods of fruits and vegetables to your meals, the pH numbers will begin to decline. This is not only to be expected, it's what you are trying to accomplish. As you continue to replenish your reserves, first your pH will drop to 5.5. After it has "bottomed out," the pH will begin to climb. It may take weeks or months for this to happen, but, in time, you will be able to see evidence that your reserves are building.

What happens is that organic sodium becomes available to work with the buffer systems we talk about in Chapter 15 to neutralize acids. As your reserves are replenished, enough sodium will be available for the urine to be eliminated in an alkaline state. When you begin eating mostly alkaline ash foods, you will be *getting better* as your urine pH drops from 7.0 to 6.4 and 5.5. You will be *getting healthy* when you are eating predominantly alkaline ash foods and your urine pH begins to rise to 6.4 and 7.0. You can re-check your progress by occasionally trying a day of nothing but acid ash foods to see if the numbers drop.

WELLNESS PRINCIPLE: *You are healthy if your morning urine pH is 5.5 after eating meats, eggs, bread, milk, cheese, and cereals the day before.*

Monitoring pH doesn't bring only bad news, and everyone isn't running around with low sodium levels. If your urine pH on Day One was above 6.0 and it went below 6.0 after acid ash days, you are probably asymptomatic. Even better than that, you now know that your body is still able to handle the protein you are eating. If you passed this test, the more alkaline ash foods you eat, the higher your pH will go. But don't get too cocky or complacent. Remember, disease doesn't develop overnight. Our diets lay the groundwork for disease years before symptoms appear. If you are in your twenties and you ate reasonable quantities of vegetables under your mother's watchful eye, but now that you are "grown" you "forget" to include vegetables in your daily fare, you just haven't had enough time to go through your alkaline reserve completely. Now is the time to fortify your alkaline reserve by including a couple of extra portions of vegetables and fruits in your diet every day.

WHAT YOUR SALIVA pH READINGS MEAN

Now for a look at what you can learn from saliva pH. Saliva pH indicates the pH levels of most of your body fluids. The magic number for saliva is 6.2. Ideally, your saliva readings should never be below 6.8. However, given the overall low level of health in our country, we will consider first morning saliva pH 6.2 or above as "normal." The "natural" reading is pH 6.8, but since most of the population is already sick, the "normal" is lower than that.

The most significant indicator of the saliva pH test is whether or not there is a dramatic change in pH before and after a meal, or before and after the lemon test. When your body still has enough vitality to respond to the emergency of eating (or to the more intense emergency of highly acid lemon juice), you know that you haven't reached the ultimate crisis level.

HEALTH INDEX SCORECARD
According to your saliva pH

Saliva pH Goes Up After Meal

Before Meal	After Meal		
6.8	8.0 or Higher	Ideal	Natural physiological function
6.2	Higher	Good	Mineral reserves available
5.5	Higher	Acceptable	Some reserves available

Any increase in pH after eating shows the body is still functioning "Naturally." It may be losing ground, but right now, it still has mineral reserves available.

Saliva pH Stays the Same After Meal		
Before Meal	After Meal	
5.5 - 5.8	No Change	Body extremely acid— inadequate reserves
Saliva pH Goes Down After Meal		
Before Meal	After Meal	
Any Number	Lower	pH response distorted by emotions that affect physiology

The saliva pH of most Americans registers around 5.5 to 6.0 before meals. If yours is in this range before eating and it goes up after meals and the lemon test, your alkaline reserve is low, but your body is still able to meet the demands put on it by the "emergency" of eating.

Acid saliva pH readings that don't fluctuate indicate that the body is extremely acid. Extreme physiological acidity puts a tremendous strain on your body. Recall that in addition to acid from diet, your cells are generating acid all the time. Strenuous exercise generates even more acid.

If your saliva pH shows your body is already very acid, it is important that you understand that *your body may not be able to continue to function under the additional acid load generated by strenuous exercise!* Remember, any system of the body can become overloaded; adding acid generated by exercise to a body already toxic from diet may be more than the body can handle. More about acid and exercise in chapters that follow.

WELLNESS PRINCIPLE: *An acid body + excessive, strenuous exercise = disaster*

Of course, there are few absolutes in life, and saliva pH conforms to that rule. Emotional upsets can skew saliva pH numbers and give you an inaccurate picture. Your thoughts and emotions affect your pH numbers. Even upsets that occurred in the past—near or distant past—can continue to have a bearing on your physiology and saliva pH.

If your saliva pH was lower after eating than the pH before, you were getting a distorted reading: emotions, or Thoughts, were dominating your physiology even before you ate anything.

Occasionally I have a patient who for months diligently follows the dietary patterns set forth in this book, yet his pH numbers don't improve. His urine pH indicates adequate reserve minerals, but his saliva pH simply will not rise to the occasion. In these cases, I know that some stimulus other than diet is controlling his physiology.

We know that the body is an integrated entity and that activity in one cell or part of the body affects all other cells or parts of the body. Saliva pH that stays around 6.0 even though the diet is made up mostly of alkaline ash foods indicates that overall toxicity is not a problem—Thoughts are involved. Thoughts are the principal acid generators for the body.

WELLNESS PRINCIPLE: *Negative Thoughts = "Acid Thoughts" = Disease*

Those whose emotional lives are stuck on anger, frustration, fear, resentment, or other negative attitudes live in a continuous mode of physiological defense, whether they are aware of it or not. They are under unrelenting internal stress. They don't relax even when they're asleep. During sleep, physiology is run exclusively by the subconscious mind; the body is on automatic pilot. If a person is so stressed-out that his physiological processes are in overdrive while he is sleeping, his saliva pH numbers will show it.

Many times, the stress has been brought about by incidents or perceptions of the past: subconscious memories that have been completely put out of the conscious mind. This stress physiology dramatically influences how the body functions. The person may not be visibly defensive, but he is internally defensive.

Findings from comprehensive health classes held at my clinic show that improving the diet will make little, if any, difference in saliva pH readings of those who are constantly uptight. But that's another whole book.

> **WELLNESS PRINCIPLE:** *Diet is a major factor in health–but not the only one.*

CHAPTER 13

Your Magnificent Cells

The primary purpose of checking the pH of body fluids is to find out if your cells are living in comfortable surroundings. Since we live or die at the cellular level, the neighborhood where our cells carry out their life-sustaining activities needs to be ecologically sound.

With the advent of the high-powered electron microscope, the internal structure of cells can be seen in greater detail than ever before. Areas that at one time were thought to be gelatin-like masses can be seen to be intricate networks of structures vital to cell activity.

Cells are busy little rascals. The level of activity that takes place inside the cell membrane could rival the frenzy on the floor of the New York Stock Exchange on a day of active trading.

This chapter is a quick survey of cell architecture to give you an idea of what goes on in the tiny intracellular universe.

Cells come in different sizes and shapes to do different jobs. Yet in their overall chemical composition, all cells resemble one another. After all, they are "descendants" of the original one-cell ovum.

Individual cells make up tissue; tissue forms organs; and organs comprise systems. Although each cell is basically a specialized universe in itself, each works in concert with all other cells that make up the different parts of the body. The body has been described as "a social order of about 75 trillion cells organized into different functional structures. . . ."[1] Healthy, properly functioning cells work in harmony with all of the organs and systems to maintain the smooth-running

108

state we call homeostasis. When all body systems hum along smoothly with each of the many components working naturally, we are in a state of physiological equilibrium—homeostasis.

> **WELLNESS PRINCIPLE:** *Each cell benefits by and contributes to the homeostatic good of the whole body.*

Homeostasis can be thought of as a condition of physiological balance. The body is designed to operate smoothly and efficiently. The circulatory system, respiratory system, gastrointestinal tract, liver, musculoskeletal system, elimination system, nervous system are all team-players working for internal balance and for the good of the whole. Even the reproductive system is seen by some to be equilibrium oriented; it assures continuity of the life of the species.

Homeostasis doesn't depend exclusively on "loyalty" of the individual parts to work for the common good. Control systems monitor and regulate functioning systems. Carbon dioxide levels are controlled by the respiratory system in association with the nervous system, and glucose concentrations are regulated by the liver and pancreas. The kidneys keep hydrogen, sodium, potassium, phosphate, and other ions in proper proportions. There is even a system for regulating the oxygen level. All of these systems and organs need to be comprised of healthy, well-fed cells in order to carry out their individual jobs in the most efficient, healthful manner.

The two most prevalent substances inside cells are water and protein. About seventy-five to eighty percent of cell mass is water. About ten to twenty percent is *protein*. While we generally think of protein as muscle (or steak for dinner), most of the protein in your body is inside the cell. Enzyme proteins spark much of the action in cells. *Enzymes are complex proteins* that bring about chemical changes in other substances. Protein also makes up much of the external cell membrane and the internal membrane that lines all of the cell's structures.

> **WELLNESS PRINCIPLE:** *Protein is vital to cells and life.*

It may appear contradictory to emphasize the importance of protein since this book focuses on the concept that foods high in protein can be the root cause of disease. It must be clearly understood that protein is essential to health—*excess* dietary protein causes problems. You must consume protein to stay alive just as you must drink water to stay alive. However, *too much* of either can put serious physiological stress on your body and make you sick!

In addition to water and protein inside the cell, there are organs (we might think of them as machinery) to carry out particular functions. Some of these organs will be described briefly, others merely mentioned. First, a short survey of our cells' habitat.

Cells live in a fluid environment. About two-thirds of body fluids are outside the cells. Fluid outside the cells is called, logically enough, extracellular fluid. Extracellular fluid makes up *the body's internal environment*. Extracellular fluid is the vehicle that transports various substances throughout the body and to the cells. Extracellular fluid harbors a lot of sodium chloride and bicarbonate ions, but not much potassium, calcium, and other ions. (Ions are atoms or groups of atoms that carry either a positive or negative electrical charge.) Extracellular fluid also contains nutrients such as glucose, fatty acids and amino acids, and oxygen ions. With proper nutrients available to them in their extracellular fluid home, cells can survive indefinitely.

However, in order to survive and to function at their best, your cells need to be properly fed. So the question arises: How does the food we eat get into cells?

WELLNESS PRINCIPLE: *Nourishment of your cells begins with the food you eat.*

Enzymes break down chewed food more and more and more until, finally, the particles are absorbed from the gastrointestinal tract into extracellular fluids which include blood plasma. The sole purpose of digestion is to get usable raw materials to the cells. When the elements of the food are completely broken down they are transported in the extracellular fluid and can be taken into the cells. There are three ways for substances to be incorporated into cells: diffusion, active transport, and endocytosis. These methods are much more interesting and the principles more easily understood than their names might indicate.

Substances are diffused into a cell either through pores in the cell membrane or through the membrane itself. We might term this the "trickle in" system. Other substances that need a "push" through the cell membrane are actively transported with the help of enzymes or "special protein carriers." They, too, go through the cell membrane. In the third and most fascinating method, endocytosis, the cell membrane actively participates in taking in substances that become attached to it. The membrane surrounds the particle along with some of the extracellular fluid, and incorporates it into the cell. This technique brings to mind the video game in which little "men" "gulp" hapless victims.

The particles move from a fluid environment outside the cell to a fluid environment inside the cell. This fluid, not surprisingly, is called intracellular fluid. In contrast to extracellular fluid, intracellular fluid contains large quantities of potassium but not much sodium. It also contains magnesium, and phosphate ions.

WELLNESS PRINCIPLE: *We are awash with fluid—both inside and outside our cells.*

At the risk of oversimplifying, you can liken a single cell to an individual. It eats, processes what it takes in, eliminates waste, and performs the function for which it is best suited. Inside the cell are "organs" called organelles that handle specific functions. The cell membrane is also an organelle. Some other organelles vital to cell operation are the lysosomes, Golgi apparatus, centrioles, and cilia. You don't necessarily have to incorporate most of these terms into your vocabulary; the point is that cells are extremely complex, highly specialized, ingeniously engineered microcosms of life. Cells hold our lives in their figurative hands. If they live, we live; if enough of them die simultaneously, we die.

All of the cells' substances and organelles have specific functions. Since my purpose here is to emphasize the intricacies of cell workings and how the food you eat impacts the function of cells, I will talk about only a few of the many currently known organelles.

The boundaries of the cell are defined by the cell membrane—its "skin." This membrane is more than just a covering to hold the fluid and inner parts together. As we have already seen by its role in taking food into the cell, the cell membrane is a functioning "organ" of the cell, just as our skin is in reality an organ.

The fluid portion inside the cell membrane, known as cytosol, contains dissolved proteins, electrolytes, glucose, cholesterol, and esterified fatty acids. Some of the other constituents inside the cell are enzymes and internally produced waste products such as urea and uric acid. (The significance of these waste products will become more apparent later in discussions of how excess protein leads to disease.)

Just below the cell membrane is an area of protein microfilaments, called the cortex (or ectoplasm), that provides structural support.

An interconnected network of canal-like structures runs throughout the cell. This network is called the endoplasmic reticulum. The walls of the canals are similar in structure to the cell membrane. The endoplasmic reticulum connects all areas of the cell from the outer membrane to an area between the double wall of the membrane surrounding the nucleus. Substances are transported through the endoplasmic reticulum to all parts of the cell.

The vast expanse of endoplasmic reticulum membrane serves several important functions. The total surface area of this membrane in a liver cell can be thirty to forty times that of the cell membrane.[2] Some areas of the endoplasmic reticulum are smooth in appearance. These are areas where fats are synthesized and other enzymatic processes take place. Other areas have a rough or granular appearance; proteins are worked on here.

One of the most distinctive organelles is the mitochondria. Energy in the form of ATP (adenosine triphosphate) is produced in the mitochondria. (ATP will be discussed in more detail later.) Mitochondria are busy little bodies. It is in the mitochondria that glucose is run through the Kreb's cycle (also called the citric acid cycle or the tricarboxylic acid cycle). During this cycle, acid (in the form of easily eliminated carbonic acid) is produced; and the cycle goes on continuously.

Even portions of fats are processed through Kreb's cycle. They first must be metabolized to fatty acids through a highly complex process. Some molecules formed from fatty acids go through Kreb's cycle to form citric acid and, ultimately, carbon dioxide and hydrogen. We get twice as much energy from fats (9 kcal. per gram) as we do from protein or carbohydrates (4 kcal. per gram).[3]

Acid produced in Kreb's cycle can be eliminated through the lungs. However, the faster cells function, the more acid they produce. If the whole body is overly acid to begin with, this "naturally produced" acid may increase the overall acid level beyond the body's tolerance.

> **WELLNESS PRINCIPLE:** *Your body produces acid*
> *continuously.*

Many minerals, vitamins and hormones are necessary for Kreb's cycle to function in the mitochondria. If there is a deficiency of any needed element and a back-up system doesn't kick in, the cycle will shut down and the cell can die. The need for balance among the substances that are involved in Kreb's cycle is one of the things that makes white sugar and its "empty calories" so detrimental to the body.

White sugar doesn't have any of the sodium, potassium, calcium, magnesium, B vitamins or hormones that are essential for the systems to work, yet it provides an abundance of glucose. There's a lot of glucose but none of the other substances the body uses to turn the glucose into energy. As a result, the system becomes lopsided. For instance, the cycle needs a certain balance of glucose, B vitamin, and minerals. Let's say it takes one unit of glucose, one of B vitamin, and one of calcium to function—1:1:1. The B vitamin and calcium are ready and waiting, but when nutrient-free white sugar is added, the proportions are upset. Instead of proportions of 1:1:1, there will be nine units of glucose to one B vitamin and one calcium—9:1:1. The system isn't going to function; it has an overabundance of glucose. Too much of one element creates a deficiency of others.

Balance in the body is essential. In order for the mitochondria to carry out their responsibilities, they need an ample amount of the proper nutrients.

Cells couldn't function without mitochondria, often referred to as the "powerhouses" of cells. Without them, energy production in the cells would be cut by ninety-five percent.[4]

Kreb's cycle is only one step in the degradation process of glucose. The cycle generates a constant supply of acid but only small quantities of energy-producing ATP. Approximately ninety percent of ATP is produced in the mitochondria by another phase of glucose degradation called oxidative phosphorylation. This process in the mitochondria is controlled by enzymes and results in the oxidation of hydrogen ions that had been released in earlier stages of glucose metabolism.

Each cell, with the exception of mature red blood cells, has many mitochondria. Some have fewer than a hundred, others several thousand. Mitochondria are strategically located throughout the cytoplasm in the areas where energy is needed most.

Mitochondria are self-replicative. One mitochondrion can form others when more ATP is needed in the cell.

The nucleus of the cell is a world of its own enclosed in a double membrane within the universe of the cell. The nucleus contains, among other things, the genes and DNA molecules that determine hereditary characteristics.

The nucleus is also the "systems control" center of the cell. Although it controls all of the activity that goes on inside the cell, (such as chemical reactions and reproduction), the nucleus doesn't control *when* a cell functions. Timing is a response to electrochemical stimuli. In an effort to maintain homeostasis, all cells function as needed for the overall good of the body.

To say "each cell operates according to the needs of the overall body" as though there were a central "biometer" or "life gauge" to signal cells to turn off or on is not quite accurate. Instead, instructions come from two types of intra-body communication: (1) the communication system within the cell commanded by the nucleus; and (2) the communication that utilizes the nervous system to transmit signals between your brain and all other parts of your body.

Messages are sent through the nervous system to all organs and systems. Many of these messages originate in the subcortical hypothalamus, a small area of the brain that does not engage in conscious thought. The hypothalamus controls involuntary, life-sustaining activities. It helps to coordinate internal functions such as heart rate, blood pressure, hormone production, and metabolism in general. Through this system, information from a liver cell, for instance, is communicated to adrenal and pituitary glands or other organs. This intra-body communication stimulates cellular activity of organs and systems through hormones that are transported by the blood.

WELLNESS PRINCIPLE: *A cell serves two masters: its own nucleus and the common good.*

Different types of cells perform different functions. The function of bone cells is not the same as that of heart cells: a bone is rigid and a heart contracts and expands; a liver cell makes up some chemicals and changes things around; a kidney cell filters; and a pancreas cell secretes.

Of our 75 trillion cells, about 25 trillion are red blood cells. There are distinct differences between blood cells and the other cells of the body. Red blood cells are principally transportation specialists. Their primary job is to carry oxygen from the lungs. Mature red blood cells have no nucleus, mitochondria, or endoplasmic reticulum, but they do have enzymes in their cytoplasm and can metabolize glucose and form small amounts of ATP. Red blood cells are formed in bone marrow and live about 120 days before being destroyed.[5]

White blood cells (leukocytes) are formed in both bone marrow and lymph tissue. There are six different types of white blood cells, plus platelets. White blood cells are the body's defenders. They contribute to the effectiveness of the immune system and to clotting of blood. Some white cells seem to have "kamikaze" tendencies—they consume invading intruders and, in the process, are destroyed. White blood cells have a short, functional life span.

Most cells, with the exceptions of red and white blood cells, can reproduce themselves by splitting into two cells, a process known as mitosis. The life-cycle from reproduction to reproduction is ten to thirty hours for a rapidly reproducing cell.[6] Reproduction is a continuous process for certain cells such as the skin and blood-producing cells of the bone marrow. On the other hand, some types of muscle cells reproduce only infrequently, and others not at all.

Liver cells can accomplish awesome feats of reproduction. After surgical removal of over eighty percent of the liver, the cells can divide and multiply sufficiently to replace nearly the whole organ.

Cells of an embryo also reproduce at an impressive rate. In the process, they can change to form different body parts and organs. The entire human body begins with one fertilized egg cell which proliferates. From this one egg cell come others that alter size, shape and function to become the 75 trillion-cell body that takes us through life.

When you realize that everything you put in your mouth has an effect on the cells that are the foundation of your physical being, it presents a whole different view of eating. Eating can be fun and a socially enjoyable pastime. However, eating serves an infinitely more important function than being merely an exercise in fellowship or satisfaction of appetite. Particular foods either enhance or contaminate cells and their surroundings. Refueling your body needs to be both healthfully profitable as well as physically and psychologically pleasant.

Food tastes are acquired. We generally eat foods similar to those we ate as children, foods that are common to our culture, or foods of other cultures that are currently in vogue. In any moderate-size American town you can find an assortment of restaurants featuring cross-culture dishes such as Mexican, Chinese, Italian, Cajun, or other ethnic specialties. However, few eating establishments feature fertilized duck eggs or whale blubber. Our psychological tastes are not tuned to view these favorably. Food preferences are essentially a matter of habit and availability.

Americans did reasonably well in the diet realm until we industrially revolutionized ourselves into an era of "man made" foods. If our food isn't man-made per se, for the most part it is man-handled and abused. The more man processes, refines, adds to, condenses, or "improves" food, the less beneficial it is to your cells. There are a lot of things we can change in our lives to suit our preferences, impulses and wants, but how our cells function and what they need to function correctly aren't matters of choice.

Health is not the absence of pain. The law of nature is very simple: we were put on this earth to eat food that is grown on this earth. The more complex man makes nutrition, the more complex our diseases become. Disease doesn't kill us. We live or die at the cellular level. When your cells are healthy, you are healthy. When enough cells die, you die. Once again, for you to be healthy, you *must* provide your body with enough natural nutrients to keep your cells healthy. It's your health—it's your choice.

CHAPTER 14

The Protein Paradox

Throughout this book, I come down hard on excess protein. The key word there is "excess." Protein is good. We need it.

Without protein in your body, you would be reduced to an assortment of disconnected bones, chemicals, and minerals bobbing about in a 42-quart puddle of fluids. Proteins are the chief ingredients in living matter. They make up about three-quarters of the solid parts of your body.[1] Enzymes and hormones are primarily proteins. Proteins are essential for an assortment of activities and structures ranging from transporting oxygen to contracting muscles. Proteins stimulate enzymatic activity and they make up the structural membranes of cells. And to top it all off, they not only handle specific vital tasks intracellularly and extracellularly, they also aid in the movement of substances through the cell wall. Protein is instrumental in most of the functions of the body.

The paradox of protein is that it is not only essential but also potentially health-destroying. Adequate amounts are vital to keeping your cells hale and hearty and on the job; but unrelenting consumption of excess dietary protein congests your cells and forces the pH of your life-sustaining fluids down to cell-stifling, disease-producing levels. Cells overburdened with protein become toxic.

Excessive amounts of dietary protein cause toxicity and congestion by upsetting the osmotic balance of the cells. Osmotic balance refers to the equality of pressure between the fluids on either side of

117

the cell wall membrane. When the balance is disturbed, water is taken into the cells. This not only restores osmotic balance but also dilutes the excess intracellular protein. Dilution is a standard physiological method of coping with an unusually high concentration of any substance in the cells.

Although the additional water restores osmotic balance, it results in a symptom familiar to many—fluid retention, or edema.

When I refer to "excess protein," I am talking about the amount of dietary protein above the amount you actually need that you eat on a daily basis. We'll see later how much is "too much" in terms of grams or portions. For now, it's important to recognize the distinction between the physiological protein that is part of the cell structure and tissue of your body and animal protein that makes up your hamburger. Physiological protein is good. It is a natural integral part of your body; dietary protein in a fast-food burger is foreign to your body. Dietary protein replenishes your supply, but if you eat more than you need, the excess gets in the way of health.

Dietary protein must be broken down before the body can use it. Protein can't be absorbed whole. Proteins are partially broken down in the stomach to proteoses, peptones, and polypeptides. Most protein digestion takes place in the small intestine where pancreatic enzymes reduce it further to polypeptides and amino acids. Protein is credited with being an energy-producer. However, energy is used to digest it, and energy is needed to neutralize the excess acid ash it leaves. Protein uses more energy than it generates. It is a negative energy source. Could it be that this is the reason many weight loss diets feature high-protein menus?

Dietary protein leaves acid ash that must be neutralized. It takes more essential substances from your body than it provides. Dietary protein requires more energy to be used as it is processed than it furnishes; consuming more dietary protein than your body needs results in physiological deficit spending.

WELLNESS PRINCIPLE: *Protein is a negative energy food.*

A lot of energy is used to metabolize protein and prepare its waste for elimination. Processing any food increases metabolic activity; protein excites greater activity for longer periods than do carbohydrates.

When substantial amounts of carbohydrates are processed, your metabolic rate increases about four per cent. However, within about an hour of eating large quantities of protein, your metabolic rate speeds up as much as thirty percent. And to make matters worse, your body can sustain the increased rate for three to twelve hours. With a faster metabolic rate, energy is produced more quickly. This explains why people who are accustomed to eating a lot of protein say they feel sluggish and dragged-out if they suddenly cut out meats and other high-protein foods. The energy they get from large amounts of protein is different from the surge of "energy" they get from eating a candy bar. The big difference is that the protein takes longer to digest; consequently, the feeling of more energy from protein stimulation lasts longer. Protein doesn't increase energy—it stimulates! "Nervous energy" fidgety foot-bouncers, finger-tappers, and channel-changers are manifesting symptoms of excess protein consumption. Proudly, but mistakenly, they see themselves as energetic. In reality, they are hyper-stimulated.

Protein is second only to drugs (prescription or otherwise) as a major stimulant. Even coffee, tea, and cola drinks are weak sisters compared with protein. Caffeine drinks don't have anywhere near the stimulatory staying power of a steak. They are good for only an hour or so. Protein can keep you hyped for several hours.

Understanding the extended-play stimulatory effects of protein certainly calls into question the advisability of eating a protein-laden meal late in the evening and then trying to go to sleep. Is it any wonder two-legged, protein-stimulated "night crawlers" stalk the kitchens and TV rooms of countless American homes each night. How can anyone rest completely at two o'clock in the morning when his cells are doing the post-dinner protein polka? The body is still trying to dispatch the cheeseburger and milk shake that was scarfed down at seven o'clock. Then, if a midnight snack of peanut butter and crackers is added because he can't sleep, the restless one has a better than even chance of waking up in the morning exhausted. Although he thought he was resting, his physiology was working the night shift.

Crucial physiological functions take place while you sleep. This is when your body does its rebuilding. If it is stimulated non-stop with large doses of protein, it never really gets into its replenishment mode; it can't take care of internal housekeeping chores. You can live this way for quite a while, but sustained abuse eventually culminates in chronic disease.

WELLNESS PRINCIPLE: *Protein keeps you revved up even when you've run down.*

As more acid-producing protein is dumped into the body, month after month and year after year, sodium will be taken from the alkaline reserve to neutralize (or buffer) acid from food. Sodium is used to convert strong acids into acid salts that can be eliminated in the urine.

When excess protein consumption is continuous, the alkaline reserve is drained of sodium. Sodium and other minerals then must be taken from any available source. The body must adapt vital functions to meet unnatural conditions in order to survive. We saw an example of how the body "makes do" when we took our trip through the gallbladder.

Proteins are made up of the three elements of carbohydrates—carbon, oxygen, and hydrogen—plus amino acids, nitrogen and other constituents. Every amino acid contains nitrogen. Dietary protein requirements in the past have been set by determining the nitrogen balance, the amount of nitrogen taken in compared with the amount eliminated in the urine and feces in a day. It was by determining the nitrogen balance that the recommended daily amount of protein of 118 grams established in the late nineteenth century dropped to the 46-56 grams recommended in the 1980s. Even more recently, according to my technical advisor Dr. Robert Brown, this recommendation has been further decreased to 25-35 grams and continues to drop. In my opinion, the recommended daily requirement for protein will be decreased even further.

Animal protein contains nitrogen. Nitrogen isn't a "bad guy." We need nitrogen, but we don't need as much as we get from protein-laden diets. Your body can eliminate nitrogen from moderate amounts of protein as urea. Urea is a neutral salt formed in the liver and eliminated in the urine. The more protein you eat, the more urea nitrogen there is in your urine.

Although too much protein overtaxes the urea-producing system, the body has a backup system to handle the problem temporarily. A waste product of nitrogen, highly alkaline ammonia, is produced by the kidneys and most other cells. Ammonia is combined with hydrogen ions from excess acid-ash foods to yield the ammonium radical that can substitute as a neutralizing agent when there is a lack of sodium in the alkaline reserve. However, this is a backup system only. Ammonia as a neutralizer is an effective short-term measure for keeping metabolic acidity under control. However, depending on it certainly doesn't conform to the long-term design. For year after year buffering, the design calls for buffering by minerals of the alkaline reserve. When the alkaline reserve is depleted, ammonia as a neutralizer is a short-term solution necessary for survival.

The way ammonia is adapted to handle the emergency of long-term processing of excess protein illustrates the ingenious nature of the body. Nitrogen, a waste product of excess protein, must ultimately be eliminated as ammonia. However, before it is eliminated, ammonia can be used to neutralize the acidifying effects of the excess protein. A truly marvelous emergency system! This design feature is why you can have a high urine pH reading of 7.5 or 8.0 indicating that your urine is slightly alkaline. Although the urine is alkaline because of the ammonia, the ammonia is present because of excess acidifying protein. Urine that is alkaline as a result of ammonia indicates that you are in serious trouble.

Ammonia is very alkaline. However, alkalinity due to ammonia does not indicate a well-stocked alkaline reserve. Alkaline urine of pH 7.5 or 8.0 that results from eating fruits and vegetables is the measure of the alkaline reserve. Alkaline urine due to ammonia is a severe reaction of acidosis. Urinary ammonia nitrogen makes up "about 2.5% to 4.5% of the total nitrogen." This amount goes up to about 5% when the body is in acidosis.[2] Under these conditions, the body is so toxic that normal, natural functions have been put out of commission and the body is fighting for survival by using a second-best, "spare tire" method of handling the situation.

As still more protein is eaten, additional acid ash generates even more nitrogen. Excess nitrogen is then eliminated as uric acid, which is familiar to anyone who suffers with gout.

When the toxic load becomes so great that the alkaline reserves have been drained, the nitrogen is eliminated directly into the urine, first as ammonia, then as protein, and ultimately as both protein and ammonia.

As your body continuously tackles nitrogen from excess protein, the pH readings follow this pattern:[3]

WHAT GOES ON IN YOUR BODY	URINE pH
Sodium is taken from your alkaline reserve to produce acid salts that can be eliminated	Acid (below 7.0 pH)
Nitrogen is eliminated naturally as urea	Acid
Nitrogen is then eliminated as uric acid	Acid
Your alkaline reserve runs low	Acid
Nitrogen is eliminated directly as ammonium acid salt	Acid
Nitrogen is eliminated directly as ammonia in urine	Alkaline (above 7.0 pH)
Bicarbonate is eliminated in the urine with the ammonia	Alkaline
Calcium is commandeered as a secondary buffer	Alkaline
Protein appears in the urine along with ammonia and bicarbonate	Alkaline
Extreme acidosis masquerades as alkalosis	Alkaline

This chain of events illustrates the adaptations that anyone's body must make to process an overabundance of nitrogen. Perhaps a summary of the process will be helpful.

High-protein meats generally cause the urine to become acid due primarily to sulfur of amino acids, and phosphoproteins. Sulfur is oxidized into sulfuric acid; and phosphoproteins, phospholipids, and nucleic acids "yield phosphoric acid."[4] You can see that if you eat relatively large amounts of sulfuric acid-producing and phosphoric acid-producing protein, your urine will be acid. (The effects of phosphorus on the body are discussed in Chapter 18, so I shall concentrate here on how the body handles sulfuric acid.)

The body can handle urine that is slightly acid, but not too acid. In order for the acid to be buffered to a degree of acidity the body can handle, there must be sodium, magnesium, calcium, or some other buffering agent that can be eliminated in the urine. It may appear to be contradictory to say that you need a buffering agent for the urine to be acid. However, there must be a neutralizing substance available to buffer the strong acid to a tolerable level. Sodium, calcium, magnesium or other buffering substances of the bicarbonate buffer system will be taken from the body to perform this vital function.

Sulfuric acid is a very strong acid. Sulfuric acid must be neutralized. This is where sodium and the bicarbonate buffer system play a very important part in keeping your extracellular fluid and your urine only slightly acid.

Sulfuric acid (H_2SO_4) has two hydrogen ions. Hydrogen can be displaced by sodium. So one of the hydrogen ions is displaced by a sodium ion which yields sodium hydrogen sulfate salt ($NaHSO_4$). One sodium ion along with one hydrogen ion, sulfur, and four oxygen atoms equals sodium hydrogen sulfate salt. In this compound, sodium is alkaline, and hydrogen and sulfate are acid. This means there are still more acidic elements than alkaline elements; however, the result is an acid salt that is a much weaker acid than sulfuric acid.

When you have eaten a high-protein meal in the evening, and in the morning when you get up your urine is slightly acid, you know that your reserves of sodium are sufficient to convert the strong sulfuric acid into a weak sodium hydrogen sulfate salt. You can see that in the process of neutralizing sulfuric acid, vital sodium leaves the body as a part of the sodium hydrogen sulfate salt. The sodium cannot easily be reclaimed and used again to buffer additional amino acids that come meal after meal.

This is why you must replace organic sodium in your body by eating vegetables and fruits. If you don't have organic sodium to buffer the sulfuric acid, your body will have to utilize one of its backup systems. If the backup system is used continuously, the body becomes exhausted.

Converting sulfuric acid to sodium hydrogen sulfate salt is only one way the body gets rid of the acidifying effect of high protein.

Some of the acid is eliminated through the lungs. We said the one sodium ion replaces one hydrogen ion in that process. Where does the other hydrogen ion go?

The sodium ion that displaces the hydrogen ion comes from the bicarbonate buffer system. The sodium ion was attached to a bicarbonate ion, which is HCO_3^- (hydrogen, carbon, and oxygen). With the sodium released, the hydrogen ion from the sulfuric acid combines with the bicarbonate to produce carbonic acid—H_2CO_3 Carbonic acid is eliminated through the lungs without taking along any precious neutralizing minerals.

If we eat meat, and more meat, and more meat, and fewer and fewer vegetables and fruits, we reduce the amount of sodium and other neutralizing elements in the body. At some point, we run out of available sodium. If the body can't use the sodium in table salt (see Chapter 17), and if there is not enough physiologically available sodium or other buffers, the body adapts its function to assure that the urine isn't too acid. A backup system using highly alkaline ammonia is called into action.

Keep in mind that the body will respond perfectly to every situation. When the environment in the tubules of the kidneys is highly acidic, the cells of the tubules produce a greater supply of the hormone glutaminase that causes ammonia to be released from the amino acid glutamine.

Consequently, if you eat a high protein, acid ash-producing meal at night and there is not enough neutralizing sodium to lower the acid level, ammonia will be released to buffer the acid urine. Ammonia is highly alkaline. If your urine is alkaline when you get up in the morning, you know that your body is using ammonia to make up for the deficiency of sodium.

An alkaline urine several hours after a high protein, acid ash-producing meal shows that there isn't enough reserve sodium available and your body is using its ammonia backup system. Without this system, your urine would be so acid that it would burn cells and tissue.

The odor of ammonia in urine is a signal that the body is responding to an emergency of too little usable sodium. The odor of ammonia is usual in the rooms of patients who are in the final stages of cancer.

Sad to say, adults don't have a monopoly on this pattern. Children and babies whose diets lack sodium-replenishing foods are also affected. A baby's diaper that smells strongly of ammonia is a signal that the child's body is adapting to handle excess nitrogen.

If the baby is nursing, the mother's milk is probably higher in protein that it should be. The quality of the milk reflects the quality of the mother's diet. A nursing mother should be especially conscientious about eating large quantities of vegetables and fruits. Her baby's health depends on it. If the baby is not nursing, he or she should be fed a mixture of goat's milk, fresh carrot juice, and distilled water as described in Chapter 10.

> **WELLNESS PRINCIPLE:** *The odor of ammonia in urine is a strong signal that the body desperately needs organic sodium and that protein consumption must be reduced.*

The body adapts through some ingenious defense mechanisms to cope with just about anything we throw at it. The crunch comes with the spin-off of the adaptations. This is where your long-term health becomes involved. Nothing in the body happens in isolation; an adaptation in one area affects other areas. For example:

1. Remember our trip through the gallbladder? The sodium that should have been keeping the gallbladder bile alkaline had been sacrificed to neutralize acid from acid ash foods in order to maintain homeostatic pH of blood.

2. With sodium in short supply, calcium is hijacked from the bones and lost in the urine. Bones lose mass and osteoporosis develops.

3. Acid levels in fluids increase, which sets up a hostile environment in which your cells, tissues, and organs must operate.

4. Resistance falls to an all-time low.

5. Defenses and barriers to disease are down.

Under these circumstances, the ramifications of dis-health are unlimited. Each of us manifests different "diseases" according to his own lifestyle and genetic structure (not necessarily in that order). And as if we didn't already have enough diseases from which to choose, we are creating new ways to be sick all the time. AIDS is a prime example.

WELLNESS PRINCIPLE: *Lowered resistance invites disease.*

Disease is a by-product of lowered resistance. Lowered resistance is a by-product of an unfavorable internal environment. An unfavorable internal environment is brought about principally by putting the wrong things into the body for it to work with. The greatest of the "wrong things" is excess protein.

So, how much is "excess"?

Although authorities differ on how much protein we need, as mentioned earlier, in general the recommended amount keeps dropping. The author of one medical physiology text tells us that we can keep our protein level up to par at a daily intake of thirty to fifty-five grams. We use twenty to thirty grams daily just to produce other chemicals.[5] The question is, how much of that activity is excited by the body having to deal with excess protein?

Other authorities suggest that an adult can live well on as little as twenty grams of protein a day.[6] I believe that even this amount is bordering on overkill.

When it became apparent to me in the early '70s that too much dietary protein was keeping some of my patients from responding to treatment as rapidly as they should, I reviewed the then-current nutritional requirements. I checked the National Research Council's "Recommended Daily Dietary Allowances." The 1968 revision recommended daily protein intake of sixty-five grams for adult males and fifty-five grams for most adult females. (Pregnant and nursing females had additional requirements.)

When the 1980 revision of the "Recommended Daily Dietary Allowances" came out, the recommendations had changed: fifty-six grams for adult males and forty-four grams for most females. I was amazed that human physiology had altered sufficiently in a short thirteen years so that we no longer needed as much protein as we had earlier. Of course, recommended amounts have been consistently lowered during this century. In the latter part of the nineteenth century, 118 grams was the recommended amount. However, it didn't appear to make much difference what the recommendations were; those who had been following any of them were the ones in trouble.

To convert recommended quantities into familiar foods, a 3-ounce hamburger has about 23 grams of protein. Add an ounce of processed cheddar cheese and you get another 7 grams. One cheeseburger for lunch gives the "average male" about 53% of the 1980 recommended amount, and it gives most women about 68% of their recommended daily requirement. We haven't even accounted for about 3 grams from the roll or 2 grams from ten french fries to go along with the hamburger. Even without the french fries, one cheeseburger on a bun affords 33 grams of the daily allowance—nearly 59% of the recommended protein allowance for men, and 75% for women.

And that's just lunch. What about breakfast, dinner, or snacks? Toss in a scrambled egg and a piece of toast and you have about another 9 grams. Pepperoni pizza ups the total even more, and a handful of peanuts takes the cumulative effect to "Awful."

WELLNESS PRINCIPLE: *All food grown in nature contains protein.*

I determined that since we were dealing with natural systems, I should by-pass publications that gave roller-coaster figures contrived by man's conscious mind and look to Nature for a clue as to just how much protein we need. The most Natural food for humans is Mother's Milk.

The protein content of human mother's milk is between 1.1% and 1.5%, depending upon the authority you read. Mother's milk is also alkaline in reaction. Even when mother's milk is the exclusive food of an infant (as it should be for *at least* six months), the child grows faster and creates more new cells during that time than at any other period of his life. Infants double their birth weight during their first six months on a diet of mother's milk alone. That's a pretty good indication that Nature's Finest contains all of the ingredients necessary to sustain both life and an impressive growth rate.

Yet 1.5% protein is substantially less than we had been led to believe is required. Where did the authors of nutrition recommendations get their figures?

Recommended protein requirements have been based on studies using white rats. These creatures produce milk of approximately 11% protein. However, rats are different from people. In addition to the obvious differences, rats double their birth weight in about five days.[7] Comparisons of the protein content of milk and the period for birth-weight-doubling of other mammals show that the faster an animal doubles its birth weight, the higher the protein content of the mother's milk. Horses, for example, double their birth weight in 60 days on mare's milk with a protein content of 2.0%. Lambs take 10 days to double their weight on 5.5% protein milk, and cats double their weight in 7 days on 9.5% protein milk.[8]

We really miss the mark when we extrapolate from the protein content of rat's milk to set the standard for human protein needs.

The effect of high-protein intake has been closely examined by a number of researchers. One study was undertaken at the University of Wisconsin to determine the impact of protein consumption on calcium balance. A 1974 report in the *Journal of Nutrition* stated: "Subjects given 1,400 mg calcium suffered a mean calcium loss of 84 mg when fed 142 g protein but showed a calcium retention of 10 mg when fed 47 g protein."[9] An amazing observation: when the subjects were given 2½ times more protein than the amount recommended, they lost more calcium than they consumed; when they were given approximately 1% less protein than the recommended amount, they lost less calcium than they consumed.

The report also noted that when fruit and vegetable intake was increased by 50% at the same time the subjects were given greater quantities of protein, the calcium balance didn't improve. In other words, if you subject your system to intolerably high amounts of protein, no matter how much fruits and vegetables you eat, your body still can't function naturally.

If you eat a variety of foods, you will get enough protein. However, if your diet is built around only one product, such as that of some African natives whose diet consists essentially of corn meal, you stand a good chance of developing a protein deficiency syndrome. Realistically, most Americans eat a varied diet: a lot of meat, fish, poultry, grains, and dairy products, and a smattering of fruits and vegetables. This is exactly backwards. Your body will operate more efficiently and comfortably when you eat large quantities of alkaline ash-producing fruits and vegetables and minimal quantities of the acid ash-producing high-protein foods.

The key to improving your health is to alter the proportions of the types of foods you eat. The dietary scales should be weighted heavily on the vegetable and fruit side.

We have been well-conditioned to believe that only animal protein provides a "complete" protein. Actually, on a varied diet, you would be hard-pressed to avoid all of the necessary protein elements. Meats and *vegetables* provide most of your dietary protein.[10]

In the 1982 revised edition of *Diet for a Small Planet*, Frances Moore Lappe acknowledged she had overstated her case in the earlier edition of her book by emphasizing that animal protein is the exclusive source of complete protein.[11] In Chapter 20, we will see that many vegetables such as green beans, broccoli, and sweet potatoes also contain all of the essential amino acids of protein as well as most of the non-essential.

WELLNESS PRINCIPLE: *How much meat does a buffalo eat?*

A quick look around the farm or jungle reveals a wealth of animals that have grown to good size on diets exclusively herbivorous: horses, bison, elephants, cattle, gorillas, giraffes and other imposing creatures.

Man has the option of going either way—meat and/or vegetables. As with just about everything else in life, extremes in diet should be avoided. A true "strict vegetarian" diet that includes a lot of grains and nuts can also create acidosis problems, as we shall see in the chapter on foods. Your body works best when you include enough protein to keep all systems on "go" and enough vegetables to keep your alkaline reserve overflowing as it takes care of occasional meals of excess protein.

Remember, protein is good for you—in moderation. You are probably getting much more than you realize. When you count the grams in that juicy steak, remember to count the grams in the broccoli and bread.

Twenty grams of protein each day will give you all your body needs to function at its best without putting it under undue stress. You can't eat excessive amounts of protein and other acid ash-producing foods and expect to offset the damaging effects by eating more alkaline ash-producing foods. Without adequate amounts of organic sodium, excess protein can be deadly. Even with adequate amounts of organic sodium, excess protein can overpower the body's coping systems.

CHAPTER 15

Automatic Antacids

We're all familiar with over-the-counter antacids that reduce acid or relieve indigestion. Daily, we see 60-second TV-commercial minidramas on how particular products subdue common gastric complaints. Only a few generations back, these same complaints were addressed by drinking a mixture of bicarbonate of soda and water. The claimed purpose is to reduce the effects of "excess" acid in the stomach, and all of these medications seem to accomplish their purpose. Antacids are reputed to buffer the acid; they neutralize it or make it more alkaline to reduce "burning" sensations. Hence, the trade names Bufferin®, which is advertised as buffering the harsh effects of aspirin it contains; or Alka-Seltzer®, which implies an alkalizing agent.

Yet antacids may bring about an entirely different response than we had imagined. My clinical experience demonstrates that a deficiency, not an excess, of gastric acid is the cause of "acid indigestion" and burning. I'll explain how I come to this rather "far out" conclusion.

Over the years, I have found that patients suffering from indigestion and "that burning sensation" find relief from their discomfort by drinking a teaspoon of apple cider vinegar in a small glass of water. Vinegar is acid with a pH of 2.4 - 3.4. If the problem were an excess of gastric acid and even more acid were added, the pain should become more intense—not less intense.

130

The parietal cells of the stomach produce hydrochloric acid "of constant composition, which is practically a pure solution of HCl...." The volume may vary, but the quality remains the same. We have a tendency to produce less hydrochloric acid as we get older. About four percent of "otherwise apparently normal young adults" produce no hydrochloric acid, with "the incidence of this condition increasing in older age groups."[1]

Those who suffer from indigestion or "heartburn" are displaying a symptom of toxicity. The parietal cells that generate acid in the stomach are too toxic to function at their best; they can't produce enough acid. When you add acid vinegar, the pH drops—a normal environment for the stomach.

When alkalizing antacids are added, the pH goes up. If my conclusions are correct, when antacids are used, the environment in the stomach becomes totally abnormal. An area that should be acid becomes more alkaline. The stomach is then forced to produce more acid, not less. The body must compensate for this as best it can. The body knows best.

Even without the aid of devised neutralizers, your body has automatic antacid systems at work constantly. Each works in its own time and on specific types of acid.

Acid residue from acid ash-producing foods keeps your buffer systems fully employed. However, these systems can be overtaxed. When they are, the way is paved for the development of chronic degenerative diseases. That is what this book is all about: how eating more protein than your body can handle forces your body to adapt the way it normally works just to survive.

WELLNESS PRINCIPLE: *Acid produced by food or by cells will be neutralized.*

Buffers maintain fluid pH at levels that range from physiologically tolerable to beneficial, depending upon your lifestyle. Buffers keep your internal environment stable so your body can function. They are essential for preventing the body from becoming overly acidic or alkaline. Buffers help maintain homeostasis.

Part of maintaining our physiological steady-state involves keeping blood pH between 7.35 and 7.45. If the pH deviates from this extremely narrow range, you're in deep trouble. You can live only a few hours if your blood pH gets as low as 6.8 or as high as 8.0. The principle job of your buffer systems is to see that neither extreme occurs.

Your body will make the adjustments required to subdue acids. Even if the adaptations are counter to long-term good health and comfort, your body will make them. Remember, your body never makes a mistake in doing what is necessary to survive at the moment. It lives only in the present. It doesn't respond to the past or the future. Your body isn't interested in comfort. Survival is the only concern. Physiological adaptations necessary to maintain acceptable acid levels are survival techniques. Unfortunately, survival techniques are usually second-best measures that, if continued indefinitely, stress the body. When your body continuously adapts its functions, it is operating under stressful conditions designed to keep it going. The potent combination of adaptation and stress ultimately leads to such commonplace ailments as osteoporosis, arthritis, ulcers, allergies, or even heart attack, to name only a few. Symptoms of these afflictions are indicators that your body has been adapting its functions for quite a while. If your body couldn't adapt, when conditions changed, it would stop functioning! Disease can be seen as part of the healing process.

WELLNESS PRINCIPLE: *Don't knock disease–without it you'd be dead.*

Your body is ingenious in the ways it protects itself against potentially harmful acids. However, some cooperation on your part is required to help it do its job if you intend to enjoy a long and healthy life. You have built-in systems to eliminate the acid produced by cellular activity as well as the acid from foods. Acid produced by normal metabolic functions or exercise is eliminated directly by being exhaled. Acid ash from food must be neutralized so it can be eliminated safely.

The three major systems that buffer acids in the body are:

Lungs
Kidneys
Chemical Buffers

First, a look at how the lungs reduce the body's acid level. The lungs are a physiological buffer system, the kidneys and internal buffers are chemical buffer systems.

Your lungs handle the acid generated by cells, as well as the weak organic acid from most alkaline ash foods. Strong acid generated by acid ash-producing foods can't be eliminated through the lungs; it must be processed chemically.

Even so, the respiratory system can buffer one to two times as much acid or base as can the chemical systems.[2] Your lungs adjust your physiological pH all the time.

WELLNESS PRINCIPLE: *The breath of life keeps your acid level down.*

Covalent organic acid produced during cellular metabolism or exercise is eliminated through the lungs. No problem.

It's pretty well understood that we take in air and breathe out air. On the surface, it would appear that when you take a breath, the air goes in and immediately bounces back. Actually, only about one-seventh of the air in the air cells of the lungs is replaced with each breath.[3]

Atmospheric elements we breath in go through an intricate process between the time we inhale and exhale them. New air that goes in is separated into its elements of carbon, hydrogen, and oxygen. These elements are dispersed and used throughout the body. Waste products of cells, in the form of carbon dioxide and water, are picked up by the blood and transported back to the lungs to be exhaled. The old artificial respiration maxim, "out with the bad air, in with the good," had meaning as well as rhythm.

Carbon dioxide (CO_2) also comes from carbonic acid generated by the activity of cells and muscles. The faster cells function, the more carbonic acid is generated. The more carbonic acid generated, the lower the pH goes. Fortunately, carbonic acid is a weak, covalent acid that can be exhaled as carbon dioxide and water. Carbonic acid doesn't contribute to long-term acid build-up, and it doesn't rob your valuable store of alkaline reserve.

Carbon dioxide is also formed in the cells when carbon in food we eat is metabolized. The CO_2 moves from inside the cells into the interstitial fluid and blood and is taken to the lungs to be eliminated. Blood carrying carbon dioxide and other waste products to be eliminated by the lungs has a pH of about 7.35. It is more acid than oxygenated blood leaving the lungs, which is about pH 7.4.

The respiratory system responds quickly, but not instantaneously, to changes in pH. One to fifteen minutes elapses before pH is adjusted by respiration.

You have probably noticed that you don't start to breathe hard as soon as you start exercising—it takes a while. Neither do you stop breathing hard as soon as you stop exercising. Although the respiratory system has powerful buffering capabilities, it can't do the whole job. The lungs are effective for eliminating only loosely bonded covalent substances like carbon dioxide. They can't handle the strong, ionically bonded acids (like sulfuric or phosphoric) that come from digestion of protein.

If the lungs could buffer acid that is left from excess protein digestion, we might be able to eat all of the protein and other acid-ash producing foods we wanted without suffering the consequences of long-term disease. At the rate we consume protein, though, we most certainly would pant a lot. Maybe it's just as well that the body uses other methods of buffering some acids.

Vegetable-scorning avid protein-eaters of long-standing are already more acid than they should be. Their respiratory buffer can't get rid of the overload of strong acid that has accumulated. For them, the addition of even weak carbonic acid can temporarily inflict a disastrous load of acid that is too much for their bodies to handle. We see examples of this all too often when athletes, joggers, and others in apparently tip-top shape collapse unexpectedly (See Chapter 23). Carbonic acid has been heaped on top of inorganic dietary acids their bodies haven't been able to eliminate. With their bodies already stressed by too much acid, the cumulative effect of additional acid produced by vigorous muscular activity exceeds their level of tolerance.

WELLNESS PRINCIPLE: *Vigorous exercise combined with a high protein diet can be deadly.*

An interesting difference between the capabilities of the lungs and other buffering systems is that your diet doesn't directly affect the buffering efficiency of the lungs. Your lungs may work faster and more intensely when there is a lot of carbonic acid to be eliminated, but the way they work isn't affected. Diet, on the other hand, provides the elements your body will work with. Consequently, diet affects how well the kidneys and internal buffer systems can do their jobs. If the food you eat doesn't give you enough covalent organic sodium to assist in chemical reactions, your kidneys and chemical buffer systems work with their figurative hands tied.

Proper functioning of your kidneys is vital to keeping your acid level as low as possible. Acid ash-producing foods, such as protein, give rise to strong inorganic acids that must be eliminated through the kidneys. Strong acids can't be eliminated through the lungs. Inorganic acid from protein can't be converted to carbonic acid and exhaled, so it is eliminated in the urine through the kidneys. When protein is oxidized ("burned"), sulfuric acid or phosphoric acid is formed.[4] These strong acids must be buffered before they can be eliminated, otherwise they would burn tissue on their route out of the body. Bicarbonate and sodium work together in the blood and kidneys to buffer strong acids.

Sodium and bicarbonate are reclaimed in the kidneys to keep the alkaline reserve replenished. Bicarbonate ions are always plentiful, however, they need covalent minerals, particularly sodium, to perform their buffering function satisfactorily. If organic sodium that is lost when inorganic acids are neutralized isn't replaced by sodium-containing fruits and vegetables, eventually your reserve of sodium will be depleted.

Sodium must be available to work with bicarbonate. Both are needed to convert strong sulfuric acid to weak carbonic acid and sodium hydrogen sulfate. The carbonic acid travels to the lungs to be exhaled and the sodium hydrogen sulfate, which is an acid salt, passes out of the body in the urine. This procedure takes care of the strong acid without damaging the body, but in the process, vital sodium is eliminated and lost. When sodium is lost, bicarbonate ions are left stranded without their partners.

Yet even if sodium is not replaced, the body will continue to defend itself. We saw in the previous chapter that highly alkaline ammonia from excess nitrogen elimination is used as a backup to buffer acids that need to be eliminated. You can see why an odor of ammonia from urine is an indicator that the alkaline reserve is seriously overburdened, diminished, or *gone*.

Highly alkaline ammonia urine is often accompanied by bladder irritation and burning during urination. These painful symptoms can be relieved by drinking three or four glasses of cranberry juice a day until the symptoms subside. Cranberries are among the few fruits that have an acidifying effect on the body. Cranberry juice re-acidifies urine that is alkaline due to ammonia. In the process, it soothes irritated membranes. However, drinking cranberry juice will not prevent ammonia production. Cranberry juice provides symptomatic relief but will not eliminate the cause of the symptoms. Cranberry juice should be used only to get over the hump of symptomatic bladder pain. The only way to correct the problem is to improve the diet to rebuild the alkaline reserve.

The kidneys provide very powerful buffering, but the process is considerably slower than that of the respiratory system. Hours or days are needed for the kidneys to adjust the body's pH levels. The body's fastest buffers are the chemical buffer systems that can act in seconds: the bicarbonate, phosphate, and protein buffer systems.

Although we speak of the bicarbonate, phosphate, and protein buffers as three different systems, they actually work cooperatively. Any condition that changes the balance of one will change the balance of the others. They are all in the business of regulating the hydrogen ion concentration of the body—the pH.

The bicarbonate buffer system, the phosphate buffer system, and the protein buffer system keep the fluids of your body within particular pH ranges. The bicarbonate buffer system can neutralize acidic fluids to bring the pH back up to 6.1; the phosphate buffer system can take the pH on up to 6.8; and the protein buffer system can boost the pH on up to 7.4.

WELLNESS PRINCIPLE: *Buffers are regulatory agencies of pH.*

You might think we are overloaded with buffer systems if the protein buffers take pH up to 7.4. However, each system is specialized.

Each works in a particular environment and is effective only within a particular pH range.

The bicarbonate system works in the extracellular fluid, where strong acids from ingested substances lower the pH considerably. If you did the saliva pH test, you may have had an initial reading of 5.5 pH. If your saliva is that low, you can be assured the rest of your extracellular fluid isn't normal. If your body had enough organic sodium to keep your bicarbonate buffer system working the way it was designed, all of your physiological fluids, including saliva, would be at least 6.1 pH.

Sodium is an essential ingredient of the bicarbonate buffer system. Without adequate supplies of *organic* sodium, the bicarbonate system cannot function the way it was designed. Although bicarbonate is generally credited with being the major element of the alkaline reserve that buffers acids, bicarbonate must have sodium or another similar mineral to function. This is why replenishing your organic sodium supply is vital to your health.

There is a constant, generous supply of bicarbonate ions. However, when there is little or no organic sodium available in the food passing through the digestive system, other minerals will be commandeered to team up with the bicarbonate ions. This is where overall health becomes involved. It isn't that the bicarbonate system can't operate without sodium, the crucial point is that other minerals that have their own functions to perform, such as calcium and potassium, are used instead of sodium. The bicarbonate buffer system will work! Acids will be buffered! The question is: Is acid being neutralized (a survival technique) at the expense of other health-sustaining physiological functions?

Recall our trip through the duodenum and liver. Sodium was being taken from bile to satisfy bicarbonate buffering requirements. With the sodium gone, gallstones developed. Lack of sodium can also be the underlying cause of osteoporosis. Granted, it's lack of calcium in the bones that causes them to crumble, but why is the calcium lacking? It is being used as a substitute for sodium to carry out the buffering process. Pick a disease of mankind and you are very likely looking at a ramification of sodium deficiency. This may not be the obvious root cause, but if you follow the physiological chain back far enough, sodium deprivation will appear.

WELLNESS PRINCIPLE: *Without covalent sodium, the bicarbonate buffer will work, but less crucial systems of your body may not.*

When sodium is not available as a partner for bicarbonate, the first-alternate mineral of choice is calcium. Organic calcium has to come from someplace. Again, if it isn't in the food you eat, it will be taken from the bones. (We'll see in the chapter on osteoporosis that you can't count on milk to provide calcium for bones.) When calcium teams up with bicarbonate, it forms calcium hydrogen sulfate to buffer extracellular fluid up to pH 6.1.

The bicarbonate system sets the stage for further buffering by the phosphate system. The phosphate system works in much the same way as the bicarbonate system, except that it uses potassium predominantly rather than sodium. The phosphate system operates in both extracellular and intracellular fluid, but its total concentration in extracellular fluid is only one-twelfth that of the bicarbonate system. The phosphate system also acts as a buffer in the fluid of the kidney tubules. The phosphate buffer system can raise the pH of fluids to 6.8. However, raising the pH to 6.8 still isn't enough. So there is yet another buffer system, the protein buffer system, that can jack the pH up to about 7.4.

The protein buffer works inside the cell. It keeps the internal pH environment of the cells constant so that all of the organelles can function at their best. The protein buffer is the most plentiful and the most powerful of the chemical buffers.

To say that the protein buffer is the most prevalent and powerful of the chemical buffers may appear contradictory after charging excess dietary protein with being the culprit that causes most of our physical ills. Two separate situations are involved.

First, dietary protein becomes a bad guy only in excessive amounts. Protein is essential for life. It is acid-ash of *excess* protein that acidifies the body.

Second, protein buffers have a restricted range of effectiveness — between pH 6.8 and 7.4. They do the fine-tuning. They can't take the pH of a solution from 5.5 to 7.4. The bicarbonate and phosphate buffers must get the homeostasis-seeking ball rolling.

The steady incremental buffering done by the bicarbonate, phosphate, and protein systems is analogous to the steady incremental gear-changing you do as you zip around in your silver Porsche. Although you may do most of your driving in high gear—pH 7.4 of the protein system— that's not where you start out. You leap off in low—bicarbonate's pH 6.1—and work steadily up through the gears—phosphate's 6.8—on your way to 7.4. High gear isn't effective at low speeds. Similarly, no matter how hard low gear works, it's not going to keep you cruising smoothly and effortlessly along the Interstate at 65 mph.

Buffering acids isn't a Herculean effort for your body. Buffering systems are standard equipment on all body models. The only time problems arise is when we don't maintain the equipment properly. If we put in too much acid and don't replenish the supply of neutralizers, the system will eventually break down. It isn't a design flaw; it's a simple maintenance problem with health-destroying potential. It's *your health*; it's *your choice*. Your body will work with whatever you give it. Your body never makes a mistake!

CHAPTER 16

Taking Stock of Chemical Bonds

All foods include chemicals. I'm not talking about pesticides and preservatives. I'm talking about chemical elements that are made up of atoms and molecules: carbon, hydrogen, oxygen, and minerals. Elements are joined together to form compounds: CO_2, H_2O, HCl, $NaHCO_3$, and hundreds more.

Separating elements would be simple enough if the bonds that hold all compounds together were the same. But they're not. Earlier (in Chapter 8), I talked about loosely held-together organic (or covalent) bonds and tightly held-together inorganic (or ionic) bonds. The elements in some foods are loosely bonded; those in other foods are tightly bonded. To get the overall picture of the relationship of the bonds to foods, think back to your elementary school science classes and the "Three Kingdoms": mineral, plant, and animal.

Mineral kingdom inhabitants are inorganic materials such as rocks and sand and gold and iron. Objects in the mineral kingdom are made up of substances like carbon, hydrogen, oxygen, silicon, manganese, and a vast assortment of other elements. Elements in this kingdom are held together by very strong bonds. The scientific terms for the strong, inorganic, mineral kingdom bonds are "electrovalent" or "ionic." You can consume inorganic minerals, but your body will either store them or eliminate them. We don't have the physiological capabilities of easily converting inorganic minerals into

YOUR HEALTH, YOUR CHOICE   141

usable organic materials, but plants do. That's the beauty of plants as food.

The members of the lowly plant kingdom may not be able to compute sums or build bridges or philosophize, but they can do something that man, in his finite wisdom, cannot: they can break the nearly inseparable ionic bonds of the mineral kingdom. Plants can take minerals from the soil, break the strong bonds, and incorporate the minerals into their physical beings.

Nature combines the plant and mineral kingdoms in the presence of sunlight through the process of photosynthesis. The food we eat should come from the plant kingdom. It is the source of food that the body can utilize most efficiently. We are able to use minerals that have been processed through the plant kingdom because of the way the atoms or ions of these elements are bonded.

Once the minerals become a part of the plant kingdom, the bonds are no longer strong; in fact, they become very weak. Elements in the plant kingdom are held together by easily broken covalent bonds. When we eat the plants, our bodies can snap apart the bonds of their nutrients.

WELLNESS PRINCIPLE: *Plants "eat" the mineral kingdom; man eats the plants.*

Plants manufacture carbohydrates. Carbohydrates are made up of carbon (C), hydrogen (H), and oxygen (O). Everything in the plant kingdom is composed of carbon, hydrogen, oxygen, nitrogen, and a mineral. We can write that $C - H - O - N - mineral$. The mineral could be an element such as iron, manganese, magnesium, calcium, sodium, potassium, phosphorus, or sulfur.

When we eat plants (vegetables and fruit), the carbon, hydrogen, and oxygen are taken into the body and used for energy. When the body is finished with them, these elements are eliminated through the lungs and kidneys. The loosely bonded minerals that are left can be used to support various physiological activities: iron for the blood, calcium for bones, sodium for buffering acids, and other minerals for use in a vast array of chemical reactions.

Plants also provide other elements essential for complete nutrition—enzymes and vitamins. Enzymes are the complex proteins that stimulate chemical reactions. When plants are eaten, the enzymes contained in the plants assist the digestive system in processing the food of which they are a part. Without enzymes, food is "dead." The more food is commercially processed, the fewer enzymes it has.

I am firmly convinced that man is designed to consume primarily plants. Man's physiology is structured naturally to use minerals that have been processed by plants. We *can* get minerals, including organic sodium, in meat. These minerals have been processed through the plants the animal ate. Most of the meat served by Americans comes from herbivorous animals like cows, sheep, pigs, and deer. Unfortunately, however, the acidifying effects of protein more than offset the beneficial alkalizing effects of the sodium and other minerals contained in the meat.

Obviously, though, we eat minerals that have not been processed by plants: table salt, antacids, dolomite, potassium and other mineral supplements. We get the same minerals in fruits and vegetables, but they have been processed naturally. Our metabolic systems can use these plant minerals easily and effectively.

Most of our food contains minerals. The body needs minerals. It needs minerals it can use. That's what this chapter is about—why we can use some minerals, can't easily use others, and what determines whether we can or can't.

One of the most common minerals we eat every day is table salt, sodium chloride. Unfortunately, even though we have been conditioned to believe that salt makes food taste good, common table salt is not what the body needs. This is hardly a revelation to anyone who has had any contact with the outside world recently. Newspapers, magazines, newsletters, and TV are chock-full of admonitions to cut down on salt consumption in order to lower blood pressure and reduce the risk of heart attack. Yet the connection between salt and hypertension and heart attack isn't explained clearly. Ironically, the problem lies not in getting too much salt, but in not getting enough organic sodium.

I am firmly convinced that the reason your body can't use table salt as a viable source of organic sodium is that bonds of sodium chloride are ionic. This is a recurring theme throughout this book because it is vitally important. The sodium and chloride elements are held together so firmly that they can hardly be separated. Few other substances have as great an attraction for the ions of either sodium or chloride as they have for each other. Nevertheless, sodium and chloride are extremely active elements. It is the compelling attraction chloride and sodium have for each other that makes the sodium in table salt physiologically unusable. It is useless for replenishing the alkaline reserve.

No matter how much sodium chloride is available, the body can't use it. To use the analogy of the gasoline-powered automobile engine again, if your car is out of gas and there is none available, a tanker full of diesel fuel is useless if your car's engine can't process it.

Fortunately, forms of sodium and other minerals are available to us in fruits and vegetables that our bodies can and do use. The minerals to replenish our reserves of alkalizing substances must come from the plant kingdom. Our bodies are built to use organic substances. However, if more minerals such as sodium and calcium are used to buffer acids and replenish bone than are replaced by the food we eat, we end up in deep trouble. Our digestive systems and physiology were designed to process and use vegetation.

Here we are, roaring to the finish of the twentieth century, and we are still running around with digestive systems that were designed tens of thousands of years ago. Our digestive processes haven't kept pace with our lifestyles. But since we can't redesign our physiology, we had better rearrange our lifestyles if we want to enjoy health while we are here.

Given our relatively predator-free environment, improvements in sanitation, and comfortable living conditions, if we ate the same types of foods early man ate, presumably, like the Hunzas, we could live healthy, robust lives for 120 years or more. Covalently bonded fruits and vegetables are the foods your body was designed to handle easily with energy left over for other activities.

WELLNESS PRINCIPLE: *Our bodies thrive on whole, living, organic foods.*

The third realm is the animal kingdom. Elements in the animal kingdom are also held together by easily broken covalent bonds.

Nothing exists in the animal kingdom that isn't covalently bonded. It's only logical that we inhabitants of this kingdom should replenish our bodies with substances of similar molecular structure.

We do this when we eat vegetables and fruit. We also get organic minerals from raw meat, but neither our culture nor our digestive systems are geared to handle it now.

In recent years, a story circulated about a group of students who went to the wilds of Alaska for a school project. After they arrived, their meals included raw meat. At the beginning of the new diet, the students became nauseous and vomited. This kept up for a while. However, in time, they and their digestive systems acclimated to the new foods. The students may not have become enthusiastic about raw meat, but they learned to live with it both psychologically and physically.

In time they found that eating cooked meat upset their digestive systems. Their bodies had adapted to processing raw meat. Again they became just as sick on the "new" cooked meat as they had originally on raw.[1]

Cooking affects how your body handles food. It changes the nature of the bonds. I call this the "cooking bond," but you won't find it described in physiology textbooks.

When you heat covalently bonded food to more than 130°F, bonds that are naturally weak are made stronger. As with strong ionic bonds, heat-strengthened bonds can't be broken easily, if at all. The elements are no longer as readily accessible for assimilation.

We know from experience that we can cook meat and vegetables until they are soft, more chewable, and even mushy. Overcooking can break down the fiber in some foods, which is different from separating bonds of the elements that make up the food. Other foods can become "tougher" when cooked.

A home-style experiment can demonstrate how heat can solidify the bonds of food. Separate the white and yolk of a raw egg, and spoon some of the white into a small container. Add a teaspoonful or so of water, and stir. The white disappears. Egg white is almost pure albumin, a simple protein that is hydrophilic (attracts and holds water).

Now take some more of the undiluted raw white and drop it into boiling water. It will immediately solidify and turn white. The heat has denatured the protein—its usual nature has been destroyed and the bonding changed. This cooked protein won't dissolve in water no matter how much you stir. It has lost its affinity for water and become hydrophobic. The denatured protein may be broken down into tiny particles you can barely see, but the elements still cling together—it won't dissolve. Yet, all processing in the body takes place in a fluid medium, and elements must dissolve. Bieler's statement about the effect of cooking on protein is quite straightforward: "... *the more protein is heated or cooked*, the more its colloid [gluelike substance such as protein or starch] is changed."[2]

The effects eating cooked food had on cats were studied in a five-year project. Over 100 cats were separated into groups. One group was kept on a natural diet of raw protein food. A second group was fed cooked food such as pasteurized milk, cooked eggs and cooked meat. The group fed uncooked foods thrived and reproduced. The cooked-food cats not only developed diseases similar to those common to man—pyorrhea, liver disease, and nervous system damage—but their offspring were stunted. Ultimately this group was unable to reproduce.

The most startling result of the study came to light unexpectedly after it was over and the pens were empty. The researchers noticed a dramatic difference in the ground of the pens where the cats had been kept. Vegetation grew in the area where the cats fed "natural" food had lived. Nothing grew in the pens where the cooked-food group had been kept. The soil in the "cooked-food" pens wouldn't support plant life—not even weeds![3]

Members of the animal kingdom, including felines and man, don't assimilate cooked food well even when the food is from the animal or vegetable kingdom.

WELLNESS PRINCIPLE: *Heat alters covalent bonds.*

A word of cheer before you infer that I'm suggesting you eat only raw foods. I'm not. As with the students in Alaska, most of us aren't healthy enough to eat large quantities of raw foods without feeling terrible or being plagued by gas, at least for a while. If you want to get really healthy, you can work up to a raw food diet. But like any other program to improve health, you should take it in incremental stages. Start improving your diet by gradually increasing the amount of cooked vegetables you eat every day. Your body has been handling cooked foods but probably not a lot of vegetables. After your body has acclimated to cooked vegetables, you can begin to cook them less and less until your body can handle some of them raw.

The materials you give your body should be as much as possible like the materials that make up your body. The food you eat needs to be easily broken down so that vital nutrients can get to the cells for immediate use and to storage areas where they are kept for future use. If only unusable ionically bonded minerals are put into your body, your body adapts to the prevailing conditions. It will take what it needs from another source to keep your cells functioning. If your food contains only tightly bonded materials, your body will take the required loosely-bonded substances from someplace else. Then that "someplace else" will give you trouble—osteoporosis, arthritis, multiple sclerosis, or cancer. No matter what the symptoms are, the underlying cause is that you have been trying to replenish your cells with materials held together by the wrong kind of bonds. While you have been satisfying your appetite, you have been feeding your digestive system and neglecting your cells.

> **WELLNESS PRINCIPLE:** *Appetites are learned; digestive processes are inherited.*

CHAPTER 17

Nature Knows Best

"Low Salt" or "No Salt" are some of the magic buying inducements aimed at health-conscious food shoppers these days. These lures are found on packaged foods from breakfast cereals to microwave dinners. From nearly every health and nutrition front we are told that cutting down on salt intake will improve our health. And this is true.

The principal reason given for lowering your salt consumption is that your cardiovascular system will benefit. We are told that lowered salt consumption will reduce blood pressure that is high, or will help keep normal pressure down, thereby reducing your chances of heart attack. Still true.

Some health advisors have gone so far as to suggest that you avoid natural foods that contain high levels of sodium. This advice is based on the contention that the body handles all sodium in the same way. Inorganic sodium chloride of table salt as a scoundrel of health is being lumped together with beneficial organic sodium as found in vegetables. My experience (and that of others as will be noted later) shows that this is not a valid assumption.

As we saw in the previous chapter, "salt" and "sodium" are not synonymous as far as our health is concerned. Organic sodium is essential. Inorganic salt gets in the way of normal physiology.

147

SODIUM AND POTASSIUM CONTENT OF SELECTED FOODS*
(milligrams per 100 grams)

Food	Sodium	Potassium
Almonds, dried	4	773
Roasted, salted	198	773
Apples, raw, w/peel	1	110
Apricots, raw	1	281
Asparagus,green,boiled	1	183
canned, regular	236	166
Baby Foods:		
Oatmeal, added nutrients	437	374
Baby Foods Canned:		
Custard pudding	150	94
Fruit pudding	128	75
Beef noodle dinner	269	159
Chicken w/veg	265	71
Turkey w/veg	348	122
Bananas	29	118
Peaches	—	80
Beef	228	183
Chicken	263	96
Veal	226	214
Green beans	213	93
Carrots	169	181
Peas	194	100
Celery	126	341
Cheese, cheddar	700	82
Cherries, raw, sweet	2	191
Chicken, roasted w/skin		
Light meat	64	411
Dark meat	86	321
Cod, broiled	110	407
Cucumbers, raw, not pared	6	160
Dates, dry	1	648
Eggs, fried	338	140
scrambled	257	146
Grapefruit	1	135
Halibut, broiled	134	525
Horseradish	96	290
Kale, boiled	43	221
Leg of lamb, lean, roasted	290	290
Lemon juice, raw	1	141
Lentils, whole, cooked	—	249
Lobster, canned or cooked	210	180
Margarine	987	23
Peas, green, immature		
boiled	1	196
canned	236	96
Peppers, green, sweet, raw	13	213
Pickles, dill	1428	200
sour	1353	—
Pineapple, raw	1	146
Pineapple juice unsweetened	1	149
Plums, raw	2	299
Pork (average for all cuts, cooked)	65	390
Potatoes, baked in skin	4	503
Prunes, dried uncooked	8	694
cooked, w/o sugar	4	327
Radishes	18	322
Raspberries, raw, black	1	199
Rice, white, cooked, salted	374	28
Salmon, broiled or baked	116	443

Food		
Squash	292	138
Sweet potatoes	187	180
Bacon, cooked	1021	236
Canadian, cooked	2555	432
Bananas, raw	1	370
Beans, dried		
White, cooked	7	416
Canned w/pork and tomato sauce	463	210
Beans, green, boiled	4	151
Beef, lean, broiled or roasted	60	370
Beets, boiled	43	208
Bouillon cube or powder	24,000	100
Brazil nuts	1	175
Breads		
White, enriched	507	85
Whole wheat	527	273
Broccoli	10	267
Carrots, raw	47	341
Milk, cow		
whole, 3.7% fat	50	144
skim	52	145
Milk, Human		
U.S. samples	16	51
Molasses, cane, light	15	917
Muskmelons		
Cantaloupe/Honeydew	12	251
Nectarines, raw	6	294
Oatmeal, cooked	218	61
Olives		
Green	2400	55
Ripe, salt-cured, oil-coated, Greek-style	3288	—
Oranges, peeled	1	200
Orange juice, frozen diluted	1	186
Peaches, raw	1	202
Peanut butter	607	670
Pears, raw w/skin	2	130
Scallops, steamed	265	476
Shrimp, raw	140	220
Syrup, maple	10	176
Soybeans, cooked, dry mature	2	540
Spinach, boiled	50	324
Squash, summer, boiled	1	141
zucchini, boiled	1	141
winter, baked	1	609
Strawberries, raw	1	164
Sugar, granulated		3
Sunflower seeds, dry	30	920
Sweet potato, baked	12	300
Tomatoes, ripe, raw	3	244
canned	130	217
juice, can/bottle	200	227
Turnips, boiled	34	188
Walnuts, black	3	460
Wheat flour, whole	3	370
Yogurt, part skimmed	51	143
whole milk	47	132

*Compiled from: "Composition of Foods," *Taber's Cyclopedic Medical Dictionary*, 15th edition, Clayton L. Thomas, M.D., M.P.H., ed., Philadelphia: F.A. Davis Company, 1985, pp. 2060-2075, and *Proudfit-Robinson's Normal and Therapeutic Nutrition*, 13th ed., Corinne H. Robinson, London: The Macmillan Company, 1967, pp. 829-840.

A major premise of this book is that lack of organic sodium in the diet can lead to unpleasant symptoms that involve the nervous, muscular, and digestive systems. Many symptoms (up to and including symptoms of major illnesses) are indirect effects of a deficiency of dietary organic sodium. We need easily assimilated sodium to replenish our alkaline reserves. But we can't get organic sodium from table salt.

There's nothing wrong with the sodium in salt—it's just inaccessible.

My contention that sodium chloride of table salt is an inappropriate substance for the human body is one that many authorities may find unacceptable. But by applying a little logic as we look at the sodium content of foods as they are grown, we can see what nature is telling us. When we accept that our bodies are designed to survive on the food available in nature, the logical conclusion is that food as it is grown contains the amounts of vitamins and minerals our bodies need to function perfectly.

WELLNESS PRINCIPLE: *Money may not grow on trees or other plants, but mineral-containing fruits and vegetables do.*

Unprocessed foods—fruits and vegetables, grains, beans, and even meats—are low in sodium. As a look at the list on the preceding page of the sodium content of representative foods shows, 100 grams of raw apple has 1 milligram (mg) of sodium; cantaloupe, 12 mg; cucumbers, 6 mg; whole milk, 50 mg; beef, 60 mg; turnips, 34 mg; and carrots, 47 mg. Processed foods, on the other hand, contain much higher amounts of sodium.

We were designed to eat foods grown in nature, not foods adulterated or "improved" upon by man.

This list also shows the potassium content. You will probably notice that the amount of potassium in unprocessed food is almost always greater than the amount of sodium. Is nature giving us a hint of how our foods should be? Now look at the processed foods. In most cases, there is more sodium, or salt, than potassium. Not quite the way nature intended. Noteworthy examples of this:

	Sodium	Potassium
Green Beans, boiled	4	151
Green Beans, canned Baby Food	213	93
Cucumbers, raw, not pared	6	160
Pickles, dill	1428	200
Pickles, sour	1353	—
Asparagus, green, boiled	1	183
Asparagus, canned, regular	236	166
Tomatoes, ripe, raw	3	244
Tomatoes, canned	130	217

Just how much sodium do we need? Not nearly as much as we get each day from our bologna, creamed cheese, canned soups, or fast-food burgers. The "Estimated Safe and Adequate Daily Dietary Intake" of sodium for adults has been given as 1100 to 3300 mg.[1] Another source tells us that the 10 to 15 grams (which converts to 1000 to 1500 mg) we get daily from our modern diet "is far greater than is required."[2] You can get that much in one trip to your favorite fast-food restaurant. For example, a Burger King Whopper will give you 1000 mg of sodium, and a Big Mac 955 mg. Add 100 mg for twenty french fries and 300 mg for a chocolate shake, and you're well within the range for the day. Or have half of a 14-inch frozen pizza at 1200 to 1800 mg of sodium, and you have at least as much sodium (in the form of salt) as you "need" for the day.[3]

Not only do processed foods pour more sodium chloride into your system than it can effectively handle, they are essentially acid ash-producing. So your body is dealt a double whammy.

It's a good idea to check labels of packaged foods before you buy. The sodium content may astound you. Remember, we were designed to live in this world on the food provided by this world. Sodium chloride is indeed "the salt of the earth." However, our bodies weren't designed to use minerals straight out of the ground. When salt-laden canned and processed foods start growing on trees, they may be fit for human consumption.

Keep in mind that your body must do something with everything that goes into it. The best course of action may be just getting the substance out of the body as quickly and harmlessly as possible. As brought out elsewhere in this book, we eliminate as much sodium chloride from our bodies as we take in each day. A problem arises when your body has to "do something" with it before it is eliminated.

Your sodium-eliminating system, like your protein system and all other physiological systems, can become overloaded and overwhelmed. When this happens, the natural survival tactic is to dilute the offending material. Your body retains fluid in order to maintain a normal osmotic balance. You may have seen signs of this the morning after having eaten generous quantities of ham or pizza the night before. Depending on your age, you may have noticed you were a little puffy around your eyes, or your fingers were slightly swollen, or your shoes were a little tighter than usual. Large quantities of sodium chloride force your body to retain fluids in order to dilute the unusable inorganic minerals.

When the fluid proportions get out of balance, blood pressure goes up. The volume of extracellular fluid is determined primarily by the amount of salt accumulated in your body, and only a small accumulation of salt can cause the arterial pressure to elevate considerably.[4] Hence, "cut out salt" is one of the first instructions to those with high blood pressure.

Now, there's no getting around it, most people prefer the taste of foods that are seasoned with salt. We have conditioned ourselves to the enhanced taste of salted foods. Salt has held a position of high esteem throughout the history of mankind. *The Bible* makes several references to salt. Most of those references use salt as an illustration of the strong bond or covenant between man and God or between one person and another. Centuries ago, salt was paid to soldiers as wages. Hence, our modern English word *salary* from the Latin - *salarium*.

Besides being a seasoning to add zest to foods, salt has other uses. It has long been used as a preservative. It is used for curing fish and meat, for pickling animal hides before they are made into leather, and in water-softening processing equipment.

One of the features of salt that makes it so appealing is its stimulatory quality. Not only does salt contribute to increased blood pressure, it stimulates the adrenal glands. When adrenalin flows, we feel as though we have more energy. Salt makes your body work harder and faster. We equate stimulated energy with health. As we have become less and less dependent upon the food nature has grown, we have had to become more and more stimulated by the things that go into our mouths. Salt is a very powerful stimulant.

WELLNESS PRINCIPLE: *Stimulation comes from the outside; health comes from within.*

One of the recurring questions that arises in response to the suggestion that salt isn't fit for human consumption is, "If nature provides all of the sodium in plants, why do herbivorous animals flock around salt licks?" In his book, *Food Is Your Best Medicine,* Henry Bieler, M.D., suggests that the animals may be "mineral starved" and that the salt may be but "a poor substitute for browsing on leaves and twigs." He goes on to say that the animals may just like the taste. "Introduce a horse to sugar," writes Dr. Bieler, "then give him his choice between a sugar mash and a salt mash. He will gorge himself on the sugar mash and ignore the salt mixture."[5]

Salt can have a deleterious effect on some animals. Dogs and chickens have died as a result of having been fed small quantities of salt. After they died, their livers and kidneys were found on autopsy "to be studded with uric acid concretions precipitated by the salt."[6]

A study was reported in the late '80s comparing the effects of sodium chloride (inorganic) and sodium citrate (organic) on hypertensive men. When five men with hypertension were on a salt-restricted diet, their blood pressure was normal. The men were given supplemental sodium chloride and their blood pressures went up within a week. However, when they were given sodium citrate instead of sodium chloride, there was "no change in blood pressure after a week."[7]

The authors concluded their report with the suggestion that further studies be done "under other metabolic and environmental circumstances."[8] Could it be that chemicals respond differently in the laboratory than they do in the human body?

I believe that, in the body, the mutual attraction and attachment between the sodium and chloride is too great for one to be lured away from the other. The two elements are bonded so strongly that they can't be separated. Although we need both sodium and chloride, the body can't use either when they are combined to form table salt. When sodium chloride is in the body, the connection between the two elements is firmly fixed.

In the laboratory, a few elements can replace sodium attached to chloride. Under particular circumstances, lithium, calcium, and potassium can have an even stronger attraction to chloride than sodium. When inorganic elements are used, these minerals can easily oust the sodium and leave it available for other uses. However, the body is not a laboratory. The body uses organic elements. In the body, if there is a shortage of usable sodium, there is also a deficiency of lithium, calcium, and potassium.

You may have read or heard that we are in no danger of running out of alkaline reserve because we have a vast supply of bicarbonate ions. Bicarbonates are plentiful in bile, pancreatic fluids, and the kidneys. The adequacy of the alkaline reserve is usually gauged by laboratory tests to determine the amount of bicarbonate in the blood. Yet bicarbonate alone does not buffer acids; it is only a part of the alkaline reserve. Bicarbonate must have a mineral partner. Sodium is the partner of choice that is called upon first.

Sodium chloride can be dissolved in water into positive and negative ions. Sodium ions are positive. Chloride ions are negative. Although they can be separated, the separation is not necessarily permanent and the strong attraction they have for each other continues.

Bicarbonate ions are also negative. Bicarbonate and chloride ions are the two most important negative ions in extracellular fluid. In the material world, positives and negatives attract one another. The attraction is so strong that negative ions (bicarbonate and chloride) can be "pulled through" the epithelium by the positive charge of the sodium.[9]

When the positive sodium is joined by the negative chloride, the bicarbonate ion goes begging for a partner to help buffer the extracellular fluid. This is not the case, however with organic sodium we get from vegetables and fruits.

WELLNESS PRINCIPLE: *Only organic minerals contribute to the alkaline reserve.*

Organic sodium from vegetables and fruits, like sodium malate in apples and sodium citrate in oranges, becomes readily accessible to team up with bicarbonate. The citrate of sodium citrate can be metabolized. Citrate is processed through Kreb's cycle in the mitochondria of the cells and the resulting carbonic acid is eliminated through the lungs. With the citrate taken care of, the sodium is left free, not strongly bonded to anything, and it can be used wherever needed. Or it can be stored as a part of the alkaline reserve.

With sodium chloride, it's different. The body must "defend" itself against the tightly bonded substance. We have noted that the number one defense mechanism of the body against unusable substances is dilution. Fluid is retained to dilute salt that accompanies our food. As excess fluid builds up, the volume of blood increases, and if the person has a tendency toward hypertension, blood pressure rises.

The relationship between sodium chloride and high blood pressure has been suspected for at least sixty years, and research into the relationship continues today. Studies reported in the prestigious *New England Journal of Medicine* offer data supporting the concept that sodium chloride can increase blood pressure in some people although other sodium compounds do not. Researchers reported "... a greater increase in blood pressure among hypertensive subjects receiving sodium chloride than among those receiving sodium bicarbonate."[10]

Although the difference in reaction couldn't be accounted for, in the report it was speculated that the chloride caused the rise in blood pressure. The researchers were on the right track. However, they were looking at how different chemical components *react in the body* rather than at how *the body responds* to them.

How the body responds to a stimulus is more important than how the stimulator reacts in the body. What the body does with the food we eat is more important than how the stimulating elements react. We're looking at the same situation, but from a different perspective.

The comparison in the study reported in the NEJM was between sodium chloride and sodium bicarbonate. Since blood pressure went up when the subjects consumed sodium chloride but not when they consumed sodium bicarbonate, chloride was tagged as the culprit. In reality, it is the body's response to the stimulus (sodium chloride or sodium bicarbonate) that is the crucial point. Although sodium and chloride can be separated in a laboratory setting, we excrete as much sodium chloride as we consume. If we get rid of as much as we eat, it stands to reason that the body can't use it.

We know that the body will respond in some way to everything that is put into it, no matter whether the substance is ingested, injected, or inhaled. Physiological responses can cause symptoms. Yet the physiological responses themselves are always perfect for the stimulus. We need to consider how the body responds to stimuli such as ingested, injected, or inhaled elements, not what the stimuli or elements are capable of achieving. This differentiation is a fine but vital line of distinction.

Consider a response you may have had to a situation in your childhood:

While attending a large Fourth of July picnic, you revel in the vast array of "wonderful" food available: hot dogs, hamburgers, baked beans, potato salad, coleslaw, corn on the cob, soft drinks, chips, homemade ice cream, and roasted marshmallows. In your enthusiasm, you "chow down" on at least a little of everything—you eat your way through the day. At the end of the day, the childhood culinary delights are topped off with a watermelon feast, and you start home more than amply satisfied—you're "full."

Soon, your stomach begins to feel queazy. Then you begin to feel sick. Then you vomit. Your concerned family can't understand why you are sick and fret that some of the food may have been "bad."

Actually, after you "get sick," you feel pretty good. Your body has relieved itself of the stimulus that resulted in vomiting. The stimulus that caused the vomiting was really a response to another stimulus. Your body responded to the stimuli of too many different types of food in your stomach: some protein, some carbohydrates, and lots of sugar. Your digestive system was being called on to process too many different types of substances at once. It responded to the internal mayhem by eliminating some of the stimuli which were creating conflicting demands.

There was nothing wrong with the picnic foods. Your body could have handled each of them individually. Ordinarily, the effect of individual foods on your body would be outwardly uneventful. However, the response of your body to the combined concoction was volcanic. Laboratory analysis of any of the individual picnic foods would have shown that none contained elements that would cause physiological distress. Yet the response the body was required to make in order to maintain homeostatic balance was unpleasant for the moment.

WELLNESS PRINCIPLE: *If you don't like a response, change the stimulus.*

What does all of this stimulus/response discussion have to do with sodium and salt? Just as your body had to respond to the cataclysmal concoction of the picnic food, it must respond to salt. Since salt can't be used, your body must "defend" against it. The first defense against salt is dilution, and dilution contributes to high blood pressure.

Recall the report mentioned earlier of a study of blood pressure responses of five hypertensive men ranging in age from fifty-three to sixty-five. The researchers found that the men's blood pressure rose when they consumed additional sodium chloride, but it didn't rise when they consumed sodium citrate.

The body can process sodium citrate of this study and sodium bicarbonate of the sodium chloride/sodium bicarbonate study. Both sodium citrate and sodium bicarbonate can be broken down into their component parts and each of the parts can be used. Sodium chloride, as we have seen, remains intact and must be dealt with as an intruder. Sodium chloride can't contribute anything to homeostatic balance. As with any "intruder," it upsets the order and rhythm of the body's functions.

An article in *Reader's Digest*[11] defended salt as a much-maligned, necessary nutrient. The article referred to the results of a study indicating no change in the blood pressure of people with normal pressure when salt intake was decreased or when it was reinstated. However, blood pressure of high-blood-pressure subjects was lowered when salt was restricted, and it went up again when their salt intake was returned to the former level. We have come to expect these responses.

The same article noted other research in Israel showing that blood pressure was lowered for overweight high-blood-pressure subjects when they reduced calories rather than salt.

The conclusions of the studies illustrate how a fundamental attitude influences interpretations of data and symptoms. If you look at the body as a hodgepodge of chemicals that must be controlled, manipulated, and outwitted, your chances of reaching erroneous conclusions are greatly enhanced.

We can be thankful that our blood pressures can be elevated. High blood pressure is a perfectly natural response of the body under stressful conditions. The biggest problem occurs when the pressure is high at inappropriate times. For example, when you go out for your daily jog, after you have been running for a while, your heart rate increases and your blood pressure goes up. This is a natural, normal, beneficial physiological response. Without this response, you wouldn't be able to run very far. Your muscles would cramp so badly from lack of oxygen that you wouldn't be able to move. And remember, your *heart* is a muscle.

So high blood pressure is natural and desirable at appropriate times. We certainly don't want to eliminate the body's ability to increase blood pressure. High blood pressure is a problem only if it's sustained when it is no longer needed. When that happens, the underlying problem is one of timing, not of high blood pressure.

Salt is not the sole cause of either high blood pressure or its running-mate, heart disease. Salt may not cause high blood pressure, but it can aggravate the condition. Salt on your steak or eggs and in processed food such as cheese, crackers, canned spaghetti and the like adds even more stress to your body as it copes with acid ash foods. A constant high level of acid in the body drastically reduces the efficiency of cellular metabolism. All cells are affected. Blood cells can't take as much acid as necessary from other cells to the various disposal sites. As a result, the heart becomes enlarged in an attempt to pump blood faster.

Heart disease is rampant in this country. You don't even have to wait until you're in your fifties for it to develop. Heart disease and other chronic diseases are the culmination of months and years of the body adapting to an unfavorable internal environment. If you start young enough and do an outstanding job of mistreating your body, while still in your twenties you can develop heart disease or some other chronic disease that used to be associated with old age. Your body takes internal abuse for only so long before it begins to show signs of disease.

WELLNESS PRINCIPLE: *Disease develops; it doesn't strike.*

If we can't use table salt, how does the body respond to it after we eat it? For one thing, while salt is in the body, additional fluids are needed to dilute it. Cells become bloated and saturated until the excess fluid is shed through the urine, feces, and perspiration.

According to some biochemistry authorities, we eat "about 10 to 15 grams of sodium chloride a day."[12] "About 98% is eliminated by way of the urine," the authors tell us, "and 2% by the feces." In describing the disposition of chloride, they said: "Chloride is excreted, mostly as sodium chloride and chiefly by way of the kidneys. About 2% is eliminated in the feces and perhaps 4% or 5% in perspiration."[13] If the body could use sodium chloride, why would it excrete as much as is eaten?

One way you can tell if too much salt has accumulated in your system is by the amount of salt in your perspiration. One day during the time I was becoming seriously engrossed in the study of nutrition, I was playing tennis. I was perspiring heavily and noticed a white ring under the arms of the dark shirt I was wearing. There was also a white residue of dried perspiration on my arms. I tasted the residue. It was salty.

Soon after this incident, I went on a distilled water fast for four days. Then I went out to play tennis again to see what my perspiration looked like.

There I was, playing tennis in the heat of an Arkansas summer—100% humidity and very hot—and I hardly perspired at all. Usually, I had to wear a sweat band on my forehead to keep the perspiration from running into my eyes. This time, I hardly perspired at all. There was just enough moisture on my skin to cool me. "Insensible perspiration," or transpiration, was regulating the temperature of my body, but no liquid was noticeable. Perspiration is supposed to be a cooling mechanism, not a device to get rid of salt.

In four days I had cleaned out most of the extraneous salt from my body. However, I don't recommend a distilled water fast. Most people are too sick to tolerate such a severe regimen without major repercussions. Water fasting is an extreme cleansing process that should never be undertaken casually or without the supervision of a qualified health care professional.

WELLNESS PRINCIPLE: *Heavy perspiration is pathological— it is a sign cells are congested.*

Not too many years ago, salt tablets were given to armed forces members in tropical climates. Some people still believe they need extra salt in the summer to make up for what the body loses in perspiration and to ward off muscle cramps.

Salt is one of the most powerful stimulants for the body; it revs up everything, including the process of getting calcium from the bone. It's the additional organic calcium that has become available to the body due to stimulation by the salt that prevents muscle cramps, not the salt.

You can get organic calcium to prevent muscle cramps from other sources. If you perspire a lot and want to avoid muscle cramps, have an orange. Cut a hole in it and periodically drink some of the juice right from the orange. Two oranges during the day will prevent muscle cramps. Everything you need to ward off muscle cramps is in those oranges. Furthermore, the sodium from fresh fruit is in a form your body can use.

CHAPTER 18

Osteoporosis by the Quart

Just about anyone who has watched TV or scanned popular magazines in the past few years has seen ads that imply aging equals crumbling bones—osteoporosis. We see "action" shots of an erect, vibrant-appearing young woman. She is shown striding confidently to meet life. Instead she meets the devastation of becoming a bent, shuffling, shawled, old woman.

The implication is that osteoporosis is almost synonymous with old age, especially for women.

True, anyone *can* develop osteoporosis if the body must continuously adapt particular physiological functions to survive the process of handling excess protein. But osteoporosis doesn't have to be as certain as death and taxes.

The word *osteoporosis* means porous bones. Bones become too porous. When this happens, they break easily or break down. The minerals needed to rebuild and to keep them strong had to be put to other use. The primary mineral of bone is calcium.

We might think of bones as strong, solid structures that give our bodies form, protect our internal organs, and serve as a frame for muscles and skin. Actually, bones are more than merely a device to keep us from melting into a formless lump. Bones are living "tissue" just as the heart, liver, and all the rest of our physical body is living tissue. Bones constantly lose and replace cells. When we continuously lose more cells

161

than are replaced, bones become more porous than they should be, and they can be easily broken or crushed.

We often hear of an elderly person, especially an elderly woman, who "fell and broke her hip." Actually, it is more likely that her hip, weakened by loss of bone tissue, broke, and then she fell.

Osteoporosis doesn't come about quickly; it doesn't automatically appear with the senior citizen package of social security payments, lower bus fares and other over-65 perks. We work for years to get our internal conditions just right for osteoporosis to finally be noticeable. Be assured, osteoporosis is in the works long before calcium deficiencies show up in x-rays or as a "dowager's hump." Between fifty and seventy percent of bone material can be lost before anything shows up clinically.[1]

"Well, I don't have to worry about that," you may say. "I take calcium supplements to nip osteoporosis in the bud." Unfortunately, despite ads that tell us calcium tablets or antacids are the answer, they aren't. Calcium supplements *may do more harm than good* since the body can't use the concentrated inorganic calcium in supplements and antacids efficiently. Whether or not you develop osteoporosis depends on the relationship between the amount of acid in intracellular and extracellular fluids and the amount of neutralizing organic substances in your body. Your candidacy for osteoporosis hinges on whether or not you have enough organic sodium and calcium to neutralize the acid from the food you eat, not how many calcium tablets you take.

I have emphasized that sodium is the primary, first-called-upon mineral to buffer acid ash left from a protein-rich diet. I have described how sodium is lost through the kidneys, and how the sodium of your alkaline reserve is depleted if you don't replenish it with organic sodium from vegetables and fruits.

In an earlier chapter, I mentioned that as little as 47 grams of protein a day can cause your body to lose more calcium than you take in with your food.

Let's relate the "grams" to our standard American diet. A breakfast of 3.5 ounces each of bacon, fried eggs, and whole wheat toast adds up to about 55 grams of protein. Here it is, not yet 8:00 A.M., and you're already over the 47 gram limit, and your organic sodium may be long-gone. If you're out of sodium, your body is going to have to snatch some calcium from the bones just to neutralize the breakfast acid.

A systematic onslaught of 55-gram protein breakfasts, plus turkey sandwich lunches and spaghetti and meatball dinners, can make major inroads into your sodium supply.

As more and more organic sodium is used to buffer a non-stop stream of acid ash-producing foods, the reserve supply runs out. We have accepted that the body is going to do everything in its power to keep going. You can be assured that the intelligence that keeps us ticking has a solution to the sodium shortage, and that solution involves calcium. The solution may not be the best for you in the long run, but it will certainly take care of the immediate problem. Keep in mind that there is no long-range plan for your health future. The body's only concern is to take care of what is going on right now.

When your alkaline reserve is gone and you are on a high-protein acid ash diet, the body's immediate concern is to compensate for the absence of organic sodium. Something is needed to buffer all of the acid from the food you eat. The acid *must* be neutralized before it can be eliminated harmlessly. When you have run out of available sodium, the next best mineral to do the buffering is organic calcium. It must be *organic* calcium, because that's the only kind the body can use to buffer acid and to rebuild bone.

There are two sources of organic calcium: alkaline ash foods, and bones. Both of these sources put *usable* calcium into the blood stream. Inorganic calcium, however, is an "almost-identical twin" that can stay in the body but can't do the work of the real thing. Inorganic calcium is close enough to the real thing that it is stored even though it can't be used. It's like those clothes in your closet that "almost fit." They add to the wardrobe so it appears there is a vast supply, but the unusable items are just closet pollutants.

As unusable inorganic calcium accumulates, laboratory tests may show normal amounts of calcium in the blood, yet x-rays may show signs of excessive bone loss along with extra calcium in the rib cage. If all of the calcium were usable, there wouldn't be any extra stashed in the rib cage. It would have gone where it was needed—to the bones. Only organic calcium can act as a buffer *and* replenish bones.

Just how much calcium do you need to consume to supply your bones the amount they need? The "Recommended Daily Dietary Allowances" revised in 1980 (National Academy of Sciences—National Research Council) says that most adults need 800 mg a day. More recently, in an article in *Family Circle* magazine (Feb. 23, 1988, p. 27),

Dr. Robert P. Heaney, "the doctor who 'spurred the national calcium craze' in 1982," set the daily calcium intake goal at 1,000 to 1,500 mg.

Unfortunately, neither of these amounts of calcium—or any amount—will be enough to stem the tide of bone loss if you eat too much protein. The body's ability to neutralize the acid ash from excess protein can be overwhelmed. The amount of *calcium* you take in isn't the major factor in developing or warding off osteoporosis; it's the amount of acid ash your body must neutralize that is the determining factor.

> **WELLNESS PRINCIPLE:** *Additional calcium is not the solution to osteoporosis; less protein is the key.*

A study on "protein-induced hypercalciuria" was conducted by the Department of Nutritional Sciences, University of California, Berkeley, and reported in the *American Journal of Nutrition*[2]. The results of this study confirm that calcium intake can't be counted on to offset the calcium loss brought about by a high-protein diet.

In the ninety-five-day study, researchers monitored the amount of calcium each of six men lost in their urine. The men were on a controlled formula diet that contained "high" levels of protein (calculated in terms of grams of nitrogen) and 1400 grams of calcium. That's seventy-five percent more calcium than the "Recommended Daily Dietary Allowances" says adults need. The researchers found that the more protein the men ate, the more calcium they lost. However, it appeared additional calcium wasn't being absorbed into the blood. The abstract of the report included this enlightening sentence:

> The consumption of high calcium diets is unlikely to prevent the negative calcium balance and probable bone loss induced by the consumption of high protein diets.

The report showed that at the rate the subjects were losing calcium, they would lose about four percent of their bone calcium a year. Four percent doesn't sound too bad; but it's like gaining four pounds a year. You may be able to handle it for a year or two, but how about ten years in a row?

Scientifically gathered figures like these show that unless you cut back significantly on the amount of protein you eat, you are almost guaranteed that, over the years, osteoporosis will develop.

WELLNESS PRINCIPLE: *Osteoporosis wins the fast-food race.*

In my clinic in Rogers, Arkansas, we see evidence that older people aren't the only ones showing signs of osteoporosis. Patients in their twenties and thirties already show indications that osteoporosis is developing.

This isn't too surprising when you consider that our dietary practices have changed dramatically since the 1960s. High-protein fast-foods, convenience foods, preservatives, additives, and meals-on-the-run are all relatively recent innovations. A sixty-year old man, his forty-year old son, and his twenty-year old grandson have all participated in the "new improved" lifestyle for about the same length of time. As a result, each generation has been exposed equally to a long-term high-protein diet. Each generation is in equal danger of suffering the consequences of excess protein and inadequate vegetable intake. Daily, each generation is losing alarming amounts of calcium.

Think about your diet and your family's diet. For how many ten-year, four-percent periods have you been making sure you get "plenty of protein"?

A patient who has devoted his life to physical fitness and health confronted this question. He became quite upset with his wife of thirty-some years when he realized that the diet they had been following all that time was a prime contributor to his physical problems. His initial response was, "She did this to me." He admitted that it was a rather unfair attitude—she is an excellent cook. In addition, she had not only been eating the same foods as he had, but she had seen to it that they both had "good, nutritious" meals. But this story has a happy ending. He is well on his way to top-level health and again appreciates his wife's concerned care.

Which brings up an important side issue. It isn't my intention to make anyone feel guilty for following the traditional "basic four" diet we have been taught is good for us. Most of us do the best we can with the information we have available to us. Although "ignorance of the law" may not be an excuse in court, ignorance of nutrition and physiology is a different matter—we're not all scientists. We are at the mercy of the "experts" to tell us how different foods affect our health. If they tell us we need a lot of protein, we tend not to argue. They are the ones who "know."

It all comes back to each of us being responsible for his own health. When you realize that all of those quarts of "nature's most nearly perfect food" are leading you down the garden path to osteoporosis, it's up to you to weigh the evidence.

Let's take a look at what milk does for, or to, the adult body.

First of all, we know that milk is high in calcium. It seems only reasonable that this good, natural calcium would be just the thing to replace a dwindling supply.

"Great," you might say. "I'll just drink more milk and I'll have all the calcium I need." And you would be right that milk contains a lot of calcium.

Unfortunately, once milk has been pasteurized, the bonds that hold the minerals together are altered and the calcium may not be as usable. Pasteurization affects milk just as cooking affects other foods (Chapter 16). Even calves can't survive on pasteurized milk.

An Edinburgh researcher reported the effect of pasteurized milk on calves. Twin calves were fed similar diets. One was suckled and its twin was fed pasteurized milk. The suckled calf thrived; the calf fed pasteurized milk died within sixty days. This might be considered a fluke, but the same experiment was conducted many times.[3]

The structure of milk is changed by pasteurization. In fact, the test for adequate pasteurization is whether or not phosphatase, an important enzyme that aids in the assimilation of minerals in milk, has been destroyed.

WELLNESS PRINCIPLE: *Raw milk is the perfect food—for calves.*

We have already seen in an earlier chapter that mothers' milk is lower in protein than cows' milk, and we know that babies thrive on mothers' milk. Mothers' milk boasts other important qualities that keeps it from over-acidifying the infant's body. Compared with cows' milk, mothers' milk has a higher ratio of calcium to phosphorus, and more sodium than phosphorus.[4]

Infants can use the calcium in mothers' milk much better than they (or adults) can use the calcium in cows' milk. Human milk is produced specifically to nourish rapidly growing offspring. It provides the child with organic minerals that are ready, willing, and able to help a young body function at its best and produce the thousands of new cells needed for growth. There are enough alkalizing minerals to handle the acid from protein and phosphorus. Cows' milk (and most other sources of dietary calcium other than fruits and vegetables) also has large amounts of tightly bonded phosphorus tagging along.

We don't hear much about the phosphorus in milk. There's a lot said about milk meeting your calcium needs, but its close partner, phosphorus, is ignored.

Phosphorus is essential. I talk elsewhere in this book about the importance of energy-producing ATP, adenosine tri*phosphate*, and about the *phosphate* buffer system. We need phosphorus.

In some ways, the situation with phosphorus can be compared with that of protein. Both phosphorus and protein (1) are ingredients essential to the proper functioning of the body, (2) work in their own buffer system, and yet (3) add to the acid level of the body.

We get phosphorus—organic, loosely bonded, and ready for use —from fruits, vegetables and whole grains. This is the kind of phosphorus the phosphate buffer system can use to regulate intracellular and extracellular pH.

We get tightly bonded, inorganic phosphorus in the form of phosphoric acid when protein foods are digested. Phosphoric acid is a strong acid that must be neutralized. (You also get an extremely heavy dose of phosphoric acid from most nationally advertised soft drinks.) If there isn't enough sodium around to buffer the acid, calcium must be used.

You can see where this is leading:

- Cows' milk contains phosphorus that has an acidifying effect the body must handle;

- Cows' milk has a lot of protein that leaves an acid ash to be neutralized; and

• Cows' milk has more acidifying elements (such as phosphorus
and chlorides) than alkalizing elements (such as calcium and
magnesium).

There is about twenty-seven percent more calcium than phosphorus in cows' milk. Calcium is an alkalizing element; phosphorus
is an acidifying element. If these were the only two elements in the
milk, the phosphorus would be neutralized. But there are other elements involved such as acid-producing protein.

You may have read that milk has a neutral or an alkalizing effect
on your body. Very likely, this was absolutely correct in days gone by.
Back in the time when cows grazed on food that came straight from
untreated soil, or were fed food that was free of additives, milk had a
neutral or alkalizing effect. However, those days are gone. Presumably they will return as we become more aware of the consequences
of tampering with nature.

Milk had an alkalizing effect until the protein content of the
cows' food was increased. Higher protein content means greater
milk production. Over the years, cows have been fed more and more
protein to increase milk production. Milk from high-protein-fed
cows has a greater acidifying effect on humans. The same can be said
for human mothers' milk. As protein intake increases, the acid level
of mothers' milk increases.

WELLNESS PRINCIPLE: *Calcium alkalizes the body;
phosphorus has an acidifying effect.*

In cows' milk, there are more acid producing substances than the
meager twenty-seven percent margin of calcium can neutralize. The
small additional amount of calcium can't buffer the combined load
of protein, phosphorus, and other acidifiers in the milk. The acidifying clout of milk is just too great for the calcium it contains to handle.
However, if calcium is needed as a neutralizer for survival, the body
will get it!

The most readily available source is the bones. Calcium will be
absorbed from the bones into the bloodstream.

Calcium from the bones is in the form of a neutral salt, calcium
phosphate. Calcium that comes from the bones has phosphorus

closely attached. Calcium phosphate is absorbed into the bloodstream and passed through the kidneys, where the two elements are separated. Phosphorus is eliminated in the urine, and ready-to-be-used organic calcium is then able to help the bicarbonate buffer system neutralize acid and perform the many other important functions in the body that only organic calcium can handle.

Fortunately, the kidneys can liberate the calcium from its phosphorus partner. Otherwise, calcium coming from bone couldn't be used any better than calcium in milk.

Using bone calcium to neutralize minerals is a backup buffering system. However, if we continue to overload our bodies with excess protein, the system just can't work as fast as we can abuse it. To try to meet the incessant demand, more and more calcium is taken from the bones and the bones become more and more porous, brittle, and fragile. Osteoporosis! Let's recap this important process.

If you're sitting around with your sodium reserve on "empty," calcium will have to take up the buffering slack. The calcium will come either from your bones or your diet. Milk is indeed nature's best source of calcium, but the calcium in milk isn't up to the job in terms of either quantity or quality.

If milk were the best defense against osteoporosis, we wouldn't see more osteoporosis among people in milk-drinking countries than among those in countries where less milk is consumed. Osteoporosis is more common among the populaces of Great Britain, Sweden, and the United States, where larger quantities of calcium are consumed than in the less affluent, low-calcium consuming populations of Hong Kong and Singapore, and the Bantus of South Africa.[5]

When we drink calcium-rich milk, we are also getting large quantities of phosphorus and protein. There is a lot of calcium in milk, but it's not usable. It's rather like putting modern appliances in a house with no gas or electricity. The goodies are there all right, but can't be used to do what needs to be done.

Those who have been on the standard American diet for years will not have neutralizing minerals other than calcium to buffer the continuously excessive amounts of acid ash. To keep the acid level of the body under control, more calcium is needed than milk contains. Most buffering calcium will have to come from the bones.

So you can see how drinking milk and eating other high protein foods on a regular basis causes osteoporosis.

The good news is that the trend *can* be slowed, stopped, or reversed!

Fruits and vegetables give you the calcium and the phosphorus you need, and they build up your alkaline reserve. Your body can use the calcium from alkaline ash foods for buffering without robbing your bones. In addition, the alkalizing minerals of fruits and vegetables improve the alkalinity of your internal environment so that vitamins, minerals, and enzymes will have a more favorable atmosphere in their work place.

Mothers' milk is indeed nature's most nearly perfect food—for babies. For adults, cows' milk and its close relatives, cheese, yogurt, curds, and whey, can issue an open invitation to osteoporosis at just about any age.

CHAPTER 19

Coping With Cholesterol

More than 500 people from our small city came to my clinic recently for a free cholesterol check. I'm not sure if the information they received caused many of them to change their ways. Very likely, some did. Those whose levels were higher than those currently recommended may have modified their diets to follow more closely well-publicized advice to reduce intake of foods high in cholesterol and fat. Those who were concerned probably cut back on the amount of eggs, hamburgers, and other high-cholesterol foods in their diets—at least temporarily.

Yet food isn't our only source of cholesterol. We produce about sixty percent of the amount in our bodies.[1] We consume the rest. The combined quantity of self-produced (endogenous) and consumed (exogenous) cholesterol is more than we require for normal metabolic processes. Endogenous cholesterol production is an example of your body's self-regulating abilities. The more cholesterol you eat, the less you produce. Moderately reducing or increasing your cholesterol intake will alter the cholesterol level in your plasma by only about fifteen percent. Extreme changes may bring about as much as a thirty-percent change.[2]

You can't tell by the way you feel if your cholesterol level is too high. The only way to find out is to have your blood analyzed. I marvel that the human race has managed to survive for all these centuries

171

without individuals knowing how much cholesterol was in their blood.

Cholesterol is found in nearly all living animal cells: liver, skin, and brain cells; nerve tissue, intestines, and adrenal glands; blood, bile, and many hormones. Cholesterol is essential. It is important to cell structure, hormone production, and metabolism. It's cholesterol and some of its running mates that keep internal fluids from leaking out and external fluids from seeping in. Cholesterol in the skin helps prevent evaporation of too much fluid from the inside and penetration by liquid substances from the outside.

Cholesterol is a fat-like substance. Like other fats and oils, it doesn't dissolve in water. If you have ever tried to mix oil and water, you know that you can stir and stir and the two may run around together, but they never really combine. Cholesterol is rather like the oil.

We know that most of the fats that travel around in the body are in the form of lipoproteins. However, exactly how cholesterol is distributed isn't crystal clear. Lipoproteins are made up of water and the fat-like lipids. Cholesterol, phospholipids, and triglycerides are three of the lipoproteins currently in the limelight.

Other cholesterol stars we hear about are very-low-density lipoprotein (VLDL), low-density lipoprotein (LDL), high-density lipoprotein (HDL), and triglycerides. A brief generalization of the source of lipoproteins and the course they take in your body may help you to keep the difference between LDLs and HDLs straight.

Lipoproteins are produced predominantly in the liver as VLDLs. Current conjecture holds that a VLDL is a large "package" containing cholesterol, proteins, and triglycerides. After leaving the liver, the triglycerides in the VLDL are picked up by muscle and fat cells. Muscle cells can use the triglycerides immediately to generate energy; fat cells store them for future energy production. With the triglycerides gone, VLDL breaks up into smaller particles of LDL.

LDL continues on its way in the blood stream, contributing cholesterol to cells as needed. Surplus cholesterol, however, can attach to arterial walls and accumulate. This build-up is known as plaque. So, LDLs are "litter bugs" that drop excess cholesterol where it isn't needed.

HDLs act as the fat-clean-up crew in the blood. They take unused cholesterol back to the liver to be reprocessed or excreted.[3] HDLs are helpful litter-picker-uppers.

Using this model, we can see that LDLs distribute cholesterol and triglycerides throughout the body and HDLs pick up the strays and send them back where they came from. This is why LDLs are sometimes referred to as "bad cholesterol," and HDLs as "good cholesterol." These terms are misleading. The body never does anything wrong. The body isn't designed to produce anything "bad"—and it is designed to produce low-density lipoproteins. Once again, the problem is a matter of volume.

You want your house-cleaning HDL count high and your litter-bug LDL count low. The objective is to keep cholesterol from building up in the arteries and forming plaque. It's plaque that accumulates in the arteries. As the plaque builds up, the space inside in the arteries (lumen) becomes smaller and smaller and blood flow is restricted. When blood can't get through, stroke or heart attack is invited.

Cholesterol in the body doesn't cause heart attacks. It is excess cholesterol sticking to arterial walls that contributes to coronary artery disease.

When there's too much cholesterol in your blood, the blood gets thicker. It's like having 30 weight oil in your car engine in freezing weather. The oil can't circulate well. Similarly, blood thickened with cholesterol is harder for the heart to pump. Eventually, the cholesterol begins to get caught in the nooks and crannies of arteries. As time goes on, more of the fat-like substance builds up on the inside of the arteries. If you looked at an affected section of the artery, you would see that it is loaded with fat. We call that atherosclerosis.

If you continue to follow the lifestyle that prompted atherosclerosis, calcium will infiltrate the fat. Now we call it arteriosclerosis—hardening of the arteries. Remember the inorganic calcium from milk and calcium supplements? It had to go someplace, and getting caught up with surplus cholesterol is one of the places.

I recall an incident from my college days when we were working on cadavers. I was attempting to cut into the abdominal aorta, which is a large artery slightly bigger than my thumb. Although I didn't know it when I started, the aorta was so full of calcium-infiltrated cholesterol that it was rigid. As I put the scalpel to it, the artery cracked.

The abdominal aorta, a large artery that runs in front of the spine and is designed to expand and contract, had become so brittle with accumulated calcium-filled cholesterol that it broke like a bone!

WELLNESS PRINCIPLE: *In the body, everything effects everything else.*

As cholesterol consciousness has progressed, health enthusiasts have turned their attention from cholesterol levels in general to triglyceride levels in particular. Triglycerides are produced in the liver from carbohydrates. They are part of the fatty substances (lipids) in the blood. Triglycerides, like carbohydrates, help in producing energy for metabolic processes.

Triglycerides in the food we eat are split in the digestive tract into monoglycerides and fatty acids. (Remember, food in the digestive tract isn't really "in" the body. Until it moves through the wall of the intestine, food is merely a visitor.) As the triglycerides pass through the intestinal wall, they are re-formed into new molecules of triglycerides. These tiny new triglyceride molecules are absorbed into the lymph and emptied into the blood that is on its way back to the heart. Triglycerides are removed from the blood as they travel through capillaries of both adipose (fat) tissue and the liver.

Fatty acids can combine with glycerol to form fats. Fatty acids are released from triglycerides as they pass through the walls of the capillaries. Fatty acids slip easily through the walls of fat cells, where they are stored for future use. When more energy is needed than is provided by the food being eaten, the fatty acids are taken from the fat cells and again transported in plasma to other tissue. The "turnover" rate of fat in cells is rather high. Intricate processes involving triglycerides splitting to release free fatty acids allow the fat in fat cells to be replaced every two to three weeks. The fat you carry around today isn't the same fat you had last month.

In plasma, fatty acids combine with the albumin of plasma protein to form "free fatty acids." By now, any time you see the term *acid*, your antennae should shoot up. High levels of triglycerides not only indicate high levels of fat that can clog your arteries, they also signify high levels of metabolic acid.

WELLNESS PRINCIPLE: *High triglyceride levels mean more acid as well as more fat.*

Fatty-acid-producing triglycerides are manufactured in the liver chiefly *from carbohydrates*. We tend to think of cholesterol and triglycerides being associated with foods like meat, cheese, and eggs. Yet it isn't those foods alone that clog arteries. Carbohydrates are involved; and there's no denying we are a nation of carbohydrate addicts. Sweets, breads, pasta, cereals. These are the staff of life for most American families as either main dishes or snacks.

Fats and carbohydrates each make up about forty to forty-five percent of the diet of most Americans. A hamburger, for instance, is fat, protein, and carbohydrates. The body uses both the fats and carbohydrates for energy. Much of the carbohydrates you eat is processed into triglycerides to be converted into energy. When you eat more carbohydrates than your body can use at the time, the carbohydrates are converted into triglycerides, then to fatty acids, and stored as fat.

Several years ago, a patient whose cholesterol level was about four times as high as it should have been came to me. I recommended that he eat nothing each day except fruits and vegetables and six eggs. He wasn't overly enthusiastic about this prospect—he didn't like eggs. However, he followed my instructions anyway. An even more important recommendation was to cut out all refined carbohydrates.

In time, his cholesterol level went down, but his triglyceride level went up. After more time, his cholesterol was up, but his triglyceride level was down. His HDLs had increased, but his LDLs had decreased. On six eggs a day—eggs that are the bugaboo of cholesterol watchers—his cholesterol level was brought under control. The crucial factor, however, was reducing his intake of refined carbohydrates; cholesterol consumption was a side issue.

Certainly, I'm not suggesting here that anyone eat six eggs a day. The point of this story is that your complete diet—fats, proteins, and carbohydrates—affects your cholesterol level.

WELLNESS PRINCIPLE: *Carbohydrates contribute to your triglyceride level.*

Now that we've gone through the triglyceride, HDL, LDL routine, let's look graphically at a simplified version of how excess carbohydrates influence your triglyceride level, your acid level, and your health.

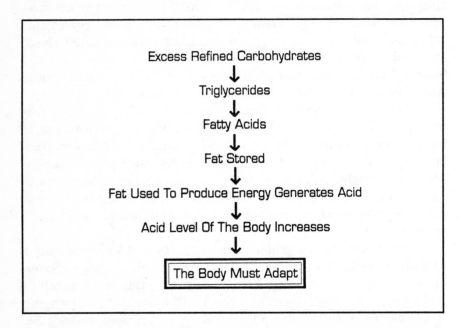

When we eat more carbohydrates than we need, even though they are neutral substances, we make acid-producers out of them. When we eat fruits and vegetables, we add health generating nutrients without cholesterol-producing fats.

There is a big difference in the types of carbohydrates you eat. Potatoes and pasta are both carbohydrates. However, they have different effects on the body. Potatoes are complex carbohydrates. Pasta is made of refined carbohydrates.

Complex carbohydrates are grown in nature. We get complex carbohydrates when we eat foods in the form in which they were grown. Potatoes, whole wheat, and whole brown rice are some of the foods that give you the fiber credited with reducing cholesterol levels. (Potatoes also are alkaline ash food that add to your alkaline reserve.) In addition, complex carbohydrates contain sugar that is held together by loose, covalent bonds. The bonds can be broken by enzymes that pick off as much sugar (glucose) as is needed at the time.

Pasta is also a complex carbohydrate. However, its ingredients have been refined. There aren't enough vitamins, minerals, enzymes, or fiber in the pasta to aid in the digestive process. The food you eat should provide at least some of the ingredients needed to help with its digestion. Refining removes most of these vital ingredients. In order for refined carbohydrates to be digested, enzymes that are already present in the body must be used, but replacements aren't provided.

Many standard American foods are more highly refined than pasta ingredients and contain even fewer complex carbohydrates. The most highly refined of our daily fare is white sugar.

White sugar is made up of two molecules that are held together very loosely—glucose and fructose. The body can sever these bonds with almost no effort. When the bonds are broken, a tremendous burst of energy is produced; your body is stimulated and your physiological engine runs wide open.

White sugar is the simplest of complex carbohydrates. Highly refined white sugar isn't bad for you; *it's too potent*. The sugar molecule itself isn't harmful; it revs up the cells, but it doesn't contribute any working materials. It contributes no vitamins, minerals, or enzymes to help process itself or other foods, but it does contribute to the triglyceride level.

Restricting your intake of refined carbohydrates will do more to lower your blood cholesterol level than will eliminating fat from your diet.

Any reduction in blood cholesterol is beneficial. Yet for those whose cholesterol level is really high, just cutting out cholesterol and fat-containing foods can't solve the problem. Furthermore, in the real world, how many of us are going to sustain a completely fat-free diet? Few of us will consistently deny ourselves simple pleasures to avoid potential problems. The "it won't happen to me" attitude is strong until a crisis erupts. Besides, plaque build-up isn't a painful process and it doesn't mar our appearance.

The good news appeared in a report of a project at the University of California at San Francisco School of Medicine. This study showed that it may be possible for plaque build-up not only to be stopped but reversed. Patients who followed low-fat vegetarian diets, exercised moderately, and stopped smoking for about a year showed a ten-percent decrease in the rate arteries narrowed due to plaque build-up. In addition, their total cholesterol levels went down by about thirty percent and LDLs were reduced by about forty percent.[4] All of the patients' lifestyle changes contributed to their improvement, and the vegetarian diet was an important factor. This book focuses on explaining *why* we should eat more vegetables and fruits, and *why* animal protein of meats can contribute to disease.

We are told to cut down on the amount of fat in our diets to reduce the amount of cholesterol in the blood. Lean meat is recommended instead. However, lean meats pose more of a challenge for your body than fatty meats. Although fats have an acidifying effect, they leave a neutral ash. Lean meats, on the other hand, not only have an acidifying effect, they leave an acid ash. When you eat fatty meats, at least a portion of the ash is neutral and the physiological acid generated in processing it can be eliminated by the lungs.

Remember, only animal products—meats and dairy products—contain cholesterol. Vegetables and fruits are your best bet for offering your body the materials it needs to become healthy or to stay that way. The body will make the cholesterol it needs from a good healthy diet of fruits, vegetables, and whole grains, seeds and nuts.

When the body is given a chance to function the way it was designed, it performs miraculous feats of natural healing.

> **WELLNESS PRINCIPLE:** *High blood cholesterol is an effect of the way your body is functioning as it responds to the foods of your diet.*

Your body uses thousands of ingredients in its natural operations. Cholesterol is just one of them. Cholesterol is having its moment in the limelight at the top of the health-conscious hit parade these days. But what about all the rest of the constituents on which your body depends? Are you sure your don't have a shortage or an excess of each of these? For instance, how about your level of lipoprotein(a)?

Lipoprotein(a) may well be the next blood ingredient we track. It hasn't yet risen to stardom, but it may have its foot on the first rung of the ladder. Researchers have found that levels of lipoprotein(a) were higher in a greater percentage of men with heart disease than in "those with healthy hearts."[5] At the rate science and technology are discovering physiological ingredients that must be factored into our health picture, we'll all soon need computers to calculate how well we should be feeling.

> **WELLNESS PRINCIPLE:** *You can't manipulate enough individual ingredients to bring about health.*

High blood cholesterol is not the cause of coronary artery disease; it is an effect of the body functioning correctly for the conditions it faces. The ingredients and chemical reactions of your blood are tied closely to all other phases of physiology. Diet is one of the primary factors.

CHAPTER 20

The Nature of Foods

WHOLE FOODS

By now you may have a better appreciation of your body's determination to survive. Your body always responds perfectly to every stimulus it receives. Every substance you put in your mouth is a stimulus that triggers precise physiological responses. Whole foods have the ingredients to spark responses that bring about more than survival. When you choose foods that serve your body best, you choose health.

Whole foods provide everything your body needs to digest, process, and use the nutrients contained in those foods. Whole foods carry with them the enzymes necessary for carrying out natural physiological functions. Mother Nature provides us with ready-made whole foods in the form of vegetables, fruits, grains, seeds, and nuts. Beef could be a whole food, but not the way we eat it. You can get everything your body needs to process beef or other animals if you eat the whole thing. If you eat it all, you'll also get more alkaline substances.

Beef in its entirety is a natural animal, but we don't eat it in its entirety. We eat the flesh. As a food, flesh produces acid ash. On the other hand, the hair, blood, lymph, cerebrospinal fluid, and bones are all alkaline. So what do we do? We throw away all the parts that could possibly supply any alkalinity and we eat only the parts that acidify us. We do the same thing with chickens. Out go the alkaline feathers, blood, and bones and we eat the acid parts—the flesh and organs.

WELLNESS PRINCIPLE: *A cow is whole food when you eat everything except the "moo."*

Perhaps you have noticed how animals in the wild eat other animals after a kill. They start with the parts we throw away—the areas of greatest alkalinity. They go for the "soft underbelly" where they get fluids and tissues that are naturally alkaline. They don't limit themselves to the muscle and try to change or "enhance" the taste with condiments. They eat their fill on the kill, and when they're satisfied, they leave the muscle for the scavengers.

So the best way to eat beef or chicken is to start at one end and eat your way through—and make sure you eat it raw.

However, there is an easier, more culturally acceptable way to get whole foods. Fruits and vegetables have all of the nutrients your cells need to keep them producing energy. Plants get inorganic minerals from the ground and convert them to organic minerals your body can use. You get the most benefit from vegetables and fruits when they are fresh—the fresher, the better. Obviously, fresh vegetables aren't available to everyone all the time. Whole, fresh, raw vegetables are ideal as the major portion of your daily fare. Nonetheless, cooked, canned green beans are better for you than a hamburger.

The ultimate in nutritious fresh vegetables are those grown in organic soil that has been fertilized with naturally occurring fertilizer, not synthetic chemical fertilizers. There is a big difference in the mineral content of vegetables depending upon the soil in which they are grown.

An article published in 1948 reported on a study of variations in the mineral content of five types of vegetables grown in different areas of the country. Cabbage, lettuce, snapbeans (green beans), spinach, and tomatoes were collected from as many as ten states, and tested.

According to the authors, "The environmental factors that seem to exert the greatest influence are soil type, fertilizer practice, and climate."[1] The report showed that the sodium content of green beans can vary from as high as 8.6 milliequivalents per 100 grams dry weight (mEq p/100 g) to as low as 0.0 mEq p/100 g, and that of lettuce ranged from a high of 12.2 mEq p/100 g to a low of 0.0. In addition, the percentage of total ash of some green beans was less than half the amount of others. This is the ash that contains vital minerals that can replenish a dwindling alkaline reserve. According to these findings, you can eat a carload of green beans grown in nutrient-poor soil and not get any organic sodium to neutralize the acid from the steak or chicken you eat at the same time.

The conditions in which our food is grown affect the quality of the product we serve at our meals. The quality of our food affects our health. Vegetables grown in an environment full of natural, living organisms are best. The question then is raised: Do I have to get all of my vegetables at a health food store? Definitely not. But you can if you prefer. Just because foods come from a health food store, doesn't guarantee that they are organically grown. The best method for determining if vegetables are really "whole," is by taste. If they are sweet, no matter where they were grown, they contain all of the nutrients they were meant to have. The sweetness test applies to vegetables as well as fruits. Zucchini, bell peppers, carrots, green beans, and cabbage are all sweet when they are properly grown. Not as sweet as fruit, mind you, but definitely pleasant-tasting and *not bitter*. Bitter vegetables lack needed nutrients. The same goes for vegetable juices. Never, Never, Never drink vegetable juice that is bitter. Pour it out. If you have a garden, pour it on the garden where it will do some good and give some future food a stab at coming up sweet.

Raw zucchini is a good example of a vegetable that you don't usually think of as being sweet. Some zucchinis are so bitter you can hardly eat them, and others are so sweet you can eat them like bananas.

WELLNESS PRINCIPLE: *Foods good to eat/are naturally*
sweet; If they're not,/let them rot.

AMINO ACIDS—COMPLETE
AND INCOMPLETE PROTEIN

A common concern about being heavy into a vegetable and fruit diet is that complete proteins aren't available in vegetables and fruits to meet the needs of the body. Anyone who has an interest in nutrition is probably aware of the advice by nutritionists and others that we need to get the full complement of essential amino acids in order for the body to rebuild and replenish itself. Amino acids are the building blocks of protein: We need protein to grow, replace cells, and repair wounds. I don't dispute that we need nutrient-laden foods; however, I believe the public has been grossly misled into believing that meat is the only food that, in itself, provides all of the amino acids of complete protein.

There are two general categories of amino acids for diet-planning purposes: essential and nonessential. Nonessential amino acids aren't frivolous amino acids that are just fun things to have in the body. Nonessential amino acids are ever-available—it's *not essential* that you eat them, because your body produces them. Essential amino acids, on the other hand, are not produced by your body. Consequently, we are told it is *essential* that we eat particular foods to make sure that we get all of them. We have been led to believe that the complete spectrum of essential amino acids is found only in animal protein.

To get an idea of what we need in the way of essential amino acids, we can look at human mothers' milk. Since newborn people grow and double their weight in six months or less on a diet of nothing but mothers' milk, the milk must have something going for it. Using the quantity of essential amino acids in mothers' milk as a guide, we can compare the availability of these same nutrients in vegetables. You may be surprised to find that many common vegetables contain as much, if not more, of essential amino acids as are in mothers' milk.

For example, look at the collection of essential amino acids shown for *Beans, snap* in the chart on the following page. Snap beans have more protein than mothers' milk, and as much or more of the essential amino acids. Only cystine is in shorter supply in green beans than in mothers' milk, and it isn't classified as essential. As you can see, all of the amino acids in broccoli and sweet corn, among others, outweigh their counterparts in mothers' milk.

Authorities differ in citing amino acids considered "essential." Most identify 20 amino acids, essential and nonessential, as being necessary to support and promote life. Yet, one source named 22.[2] In a review of eight different texts, there was consensus on eight amino acids as being essential: tryptophan, threonine, isoleucine, leucine, lysine, methionine phenylalanine, and valine. Some of the authorities expanded the list to totals of 9, 10, or 11 by including arginine, histidine, and tyrosine. One authority enumerated 8 essential, 5 nonessential, and 6 semiessential amino acids necessary for the body.[3] "Semiessential" means that the body produces some but not enough of that particular substance.

ESSENTIAL AMINO ACID COMPARISONS*

(per 100 grams food, edible portion)

Food	Protein gm	Trypto-phan gm	Threo-nine gm	Iso-leucine gm	leucine gm	lysine gm	Sulfur Containing Metholine gm	Cystine gm	Phenyl-alanine gm	Tyrosine gm	Valine gm	Arginine gm	Histidine gm
Milk													
Cow:													
Fluid, whole and nonfat	3.5	0.049	0.161	0.223	0.344	0.272	0.086	0.031	0.170	0.178	0.240	0.128	0.092
Canned:													
Evaporated, unsweetened	7.0	.099	.323	.447	.688	.545	.171	.063	.340	.357	.481	.256	.185
Condensed, sweetened	8.1	.114	.374	.518	.796	.631	.198	.072	.393	.413	.557	.296	.214
Dried													
Whole	25.8	.364	1.191	1.648	2.535	2.009	.632	.231	1.251	1.316	1.774	.944	.680
Nonfat	35.8	.502	1.641	2.271	3.493	2.768	.870	.318	1.724	1.814	2.444	1.300	.937
Goat	3.3	.039	.217	.087	.278	.312	.065	—	.121	—	.139	.174	.068
Human	1.4	.023	.062	.075	.124	.090	.028	.027	.060	.071	.086	.055	.030
Vegetable													
Asparagus, raw	2.2	.027	.066	.080	.096	.103	.032	—	.069	—	.106	.123	.036
Beans, snaps	2.4	.033	.091	.109	.139	.128	.035	.024	.057	.050	.115	.101	.045
Beet greens	2.0	.024	.076	.084	.129	.108	.034	—	.116	—	.101	.083	.026
Beets	1.6	.014	.034	.051	.055	.086	.006	—	.027	—	.049	.028	.022
Broccoli	3.3	.037	.122	.126	.163	.147	.050	—	.119	—	.170	.192	.063
Brussels sprouts	4.4	.044	.153	.186	.194	.197	.046	—	.148	—	.193	.279	.106

	1	2	3	4	5	6	7	8	9	10	11	12	13
Cabbage	1.4	.011	.039	.040	.057	.066	.013	.028	.030	.030	.043	.105	.025
Carrots	1.2	.010	.043	.046	.065	.052	.010	.029	.042	.020	.056	.041	.017
Cauliflower	2.4	.033	.102	.104	.162	.134	.047	—	.075	.034	.144	.110	.048
Celery	1.3	.012	—	—	—	.021	.015	.006	—	.016	—	—	—
Chard	1.4	.014	.058	.060	.076	.055	.004	—	.046	—	.055	.035	.018
Chicory	1.6	.024	—	.137	.407	.052	.016	.006	—	.040	—	—	.024
Corn, sweet	3.7	.023	.151	.465	.653	.137	.072	.062	.207	.124	.231	.174	.095
Cowpeas	9.4	.099	.353	.022	.030	.617	.131	—	.523	—	.513	.615	.310
Cucumbers	0.7	.005	.019	.056	.068	.031	.007	—	.016	—	.024	.053	.001
Eggplant	1.1	.010	.038	.133	.252	.030	.006	—	.048	—	.065	.037	.019
Kale	3.9	.042	.139	—	—	.121	.035	.036	.158	—	.184	.202	.062
Lettuce	1.2	.012	—	—	—	.070	.004	—	—	—	—	—	—
Lima beans	7.5	0.097	0.338	0.460	0.605	0.474	0.080	0.083	0.389	0.259	0.485	0.454	0.247
Mustard greens	2.3	.037	.060	.075	.062	.111	.024	.035	.074	.121	.108	.167	.041
Onions, mature	1.4	.021	.022	.021	.037	.064	.013	—	.039	.046	.031	.180	.014
Peas	6.7	.056	.245	.308	.418	.316	.054	.073	.257	.163	.274	.595	.109
Peppers	1.2	.009	.050	.046	.046	.051	.016	—	.055	—	.033	.024	.014
Potatoes, raw	2.0	.021	.079	.088	.100	.107	.025	.019	.088	.036	.107	.099	.029
Spinach	2.3	.037	.102	.107	.176	.142	.039	.046	.099	.073	.126	.116	.049
Squash, summer	0.6	.005	.014	.019	.027	.023	.008	—	.016	—	.022	.027	.009
Sweetpotatoes, raw	1.8	.031	.085	.087	.103	.085	.033	.029	.100	.081	.135	.094	.036
Toamtoes	1.0	.009	.033	.029	.041	.042	.007	—	.028	.014	.028	.029	.015
Turnips	1.1	—	—	.020	—	.057	.012	—	.020	.029	—	—	—
Turnip greens	2.9	.045	.125	.107	.207	.129	.052	.045	.146	.105	.149	.167	.051

*From Amino Acid Content of Foods by M.L. Orr and B.K. Watt, Home Economics Research Rep. No. 4, Agricultural Research Service, U.S. Department of Agriculture, Washington, D.C., 1957, as listed in Proudfit-Robinson's Normal and Therapeutic Nutrition. 13th Ed., Corinne H. Robinson, New York: The Macmillan Company, 1967, pp. 821, 827, 828.

More and more amino acids are being tagged as being essential. Under natural conditions, our modern-day bodies don't need any more or any less dietary amino acids, vitamins, minerals or enzymes than our remote ancestors did. The significant phrase there is "natural conditions." Today we stress our bodies by our lifestyles, including diet. Human physiological capabilities are being stretched to the maximum. Remember, the body doesn't know time; it doesn't plan for the future. It does what needs to be done to meet the situations of the moment.

The point is that no one is exactly sure what amino acids exist or are required. We have a pretty good idea, but a list of the essential amino acids that are necessary to make up a complete protein has not been sent down from on high. Vegetables have most of the essential amino acids to make up a complete protein. By eating a variety of vegetables, you can give your body all of the nutrients it needs to replenish cells, heal wounds, and have energy left over for racquetball, deep sea fishing, and other recreational or required activities.

I find it very difficult to believe that our intelligent bodies can't provide everything they need to function at their best. Our design wasn't incomplete. Any intelligence that can design perfect, intricately complex backup systems to keep itself operating under extreme conditions certainly isn't going to put out a product with missing ingredients. The only things we need to do to keep our bodies functioning smoothly are to feed them the kinds of foods they were meant to have, protect them from adverse external environments and trauma, and assure that stimuli spark only healthy responses. I am firmly convinced that when the human body receives proper treatment, it can provide everything it needs—including all of the amino acids—to function at its healthy-best.

WELLNESS PRINCIPLE: *Your body has the potential to produce everything it needs.*

VITAMIN B$_{12}$

Another concern about restricting or avoiding meats is that the body will become deficient in vitamin B$_{12}$. This important vitamin is used in the formation of red blood cells. The recommended daily amount of dietary vitamin B_{12} is 3.0 micrograms (RDA) or 5.0 micrograms[4], depending upon the information source. A microgram isn't very much. To get an idea of how scant a microgram is, divide a milligram into a thousand equal parts. Take three or five of the parts to meet your B_{12} requirement. Each of us comes equipped with about 1000 times that amount (a four- to five-year supply) stored in the liver.[5] Vitamin A comes with microgram recommendation from 400 to 1000, depending on age and sex. Of the seventeen nutrients listed in the Recommended Daily Dietary Allowances, twelve of them are recommended in quantities of grams or milligrams, which are much greater quantities than micrograms.

Dietary vitamin B_{12} comes from dairy products and from those foods we euphemistically refer to as "organ meats": liver and kidney, the parts of a living animal that take care of handling internal debris. *Your* liver has a lot of B_{12} in it too. You don't *have* to eat flesh or dairy products to get either a complete food or vitamin B_{12}. Realistically, with our current lifestyles, we are hard-pressed to completely avoid animal proteins. B_{12}-containing butter and eggs are often hidden ingredients in prepared foods.

Given the right circumstances, vitamin B_{12} may be produced in the body by bacteria termed *intestinal flora*. However, if conditions in the intestine are hostile to the producing bacteria or if your absorption capabilities are defunct because of a general decline in overall health, the supply of this vital vitamin stored in the liver may ultimately be depleted.

Vitamin B_{12} is absorbed through the intestinal wall. Even if there is a generous quantity of dietary B_{12} available, if the internal environment of the intestine is not hospitable, the vitamin can't be absorbed.

Diet isn't the only thing that can reduce both the bacteria and the serendipity of the environment in the intestine. Antibiotics can do away with both. Antibiotics are unconscionable bacteria-killers. They zap the good along with the troublemakers. Great numbers of Americans have taken generous quantities of antibiotics in one form or another during their lifetimes. Certainly, there is no doubt that antibiotics have saved countless lives since penicillin came into use in the 1940s. Yet wholesale bacteria eradication to handle an emergency situation can have subtle long-term effects. When beneficial bacteria, such as Lactobacillus acidophilus, have been done away with, the door is left open for uninvited intestinal or colon guests to move in. Yeast is one of the major interlopers that can set up shop in an enviornment where helpful bacteria are in short supply. Candida albicans, a tenacious colon inhabitant, is a common yeast that has taken advantage of the short supply of "good" intestinal bacteria.

After the bacterial "bad guys" have been routed, we need to re-store the "good guys" so they can get on with helping to reestablish a healthy environment.

Acidophilus supplementation, on a temporary basis especially after treatment with antibiotics, can help restore favorable condi-tions in the colon. "Studies conducted by scientists at the University of Nebraska have shown that L. acidophilus provides several thera-peutic effects. It has specific actions including the ability to make a natural antibiotic named acidophilin."[6] Although acidophilus has been shown to "retard the growth of Candida albicans," just any acidophilus won't do. In order to be effective, the acidophilus must be the type that can withstand the acid of the stomach as it makes its way to the intestine.

Keep in mind that any supplement or "treatment" designed to make you feel better is a stop-gap measure. Localized symptoms are warning signs that something is amiss and the whole body is affected. The condition of the intestine and colon is equally as important as the condition of the heart, lungs, or any other organ. Every cell in the body is in communication with every other cell. Trouble in one cell signals repercussions for the rest. Every morsel of food you eat causes a response by your body. No activity in or of the body happens in isolation. Taming symptoms can bring blessed relief; however, un-less the conditions that brought about the symptoms are corrected, the same or different symptoms will appear.

WELLNESS PRINCIPLE: *The body will continue to tell you that you are abusing it until you stop the abuse.*

PROTEIN

The merits and perils of protein have been discussed throughout this book. There is no question that we need protein to stay alive. The problem comes with excess. Following the premise "If a little protein is good, a lot is better" can lead you down the garden path to disease.

I talked about calcium being lost on a daily diet of 47 grams of protein. You should keep your daily protein intake under 47 grams. Obviously, an occasional binge of more than 47 grams isn't going to irreversibly damage your health. However, protein pig-outs should be limited to rare special occasions.

The magic number for protein is 25 grams a day. This amount will provide all of the protein you need physically and should satisfy the most well-entrenched psychological need for "enough protein." Keep in mind that 25 grams a day includes the protein in *all* of the food you eat, not just meat, eggs, chicken, and fish. Vegetables, breads, potatoes, and snacks all have protein in them. The 8 grams of protein in a hot-dog-on-a-bun come from the hot dog *and* the bun. Cutting down on protein isn't all that difficult. You may be surprised, after you have reduced your meat and dairy protein intake, to find that a little goes a long way.

I believe that you can maintain glowing health on a daily protein intake of the amount that is in two eggs. I really believe that you could get enough protein each day on nothing but two eggs and distilled water. There are about 9 grams of protein in a raw egg. Two eggs would be more than enough. You wouldn't have much energy, but you would have your protein supply. Obviously, I am not recommending that anyone eat this way; I'm merely making a point.

WELLNESS PRINCIPLE: *Even without meat, a variety of typical American foods will give you at least enough protein.*

You may be surprised at how much protein you eat each day. Much of it comes from foods we don't usually consider protein suppliers. For example, there are 2 grams of protein in a 1-ounce serving of potato chips and 3 grams in a 1-ounce slice of bread. Just a couple of snacks and you have eaten more than 10% of the generally recommended 47 grams.

As a guide to how much protein is in many of the foods Americans eat, a list of common foods and their protein content is shown at the end of this chapter. Comparisons of sample "good" and "not-so-good" menus are shown in Chapter 22.

CARBOHYDRATES

Although we need protein to keep our cell structure in good working condition, we need carbohydrates for energy. Animal protein stimulates us—a condition we often mistake for energy. It's carbohydrates that provide energy for the body to operate and for us to think and move around.

Plants manufacture carbohydrates. All carbohydrates are made up of carbon, hydrogen, and oxygen. There are three general classes of carbohydrates, all of which are important parts of our diets: (1) sugars, (2) starches, and (3) "unavailable" carbohydrates that include fiber the body can't absorb.

Refined white sugar is the simplest of carbohydrates. It has been processed down to the glucose-and-fructose-only stage. The body has no trouble splitting the bonds of refined sugar. Splitting bonds produces a tremendous amount of energy—your physiological engine runs wide open. Simple carbohydrates, like white sugar, rev up your internal motor by providing "quick energy"; but they don't provide the nutrients to "feed" your body as do complex carbohydrates.

Starches are complex carbohydrates. Complex carbohydrates as grown in nature (potatoes, wheat, rice, vegetables, fruit) contain sugar that is held together with loose bonds. Unlike refined sugar, complex carbohydrates come equipped with nutrients to replenish the body, and with enzymes to break apart the component parts for digestion. Enzymes can easily break these bonds, and the body can pick off as much sugar as it needs at any time. The most important difference between simple and complex carbohydrates is that your body can benefit from the more robust complex variety. They contribute to the digestive process and supply nutrients your body can store and use later. The "time release" sugar of complex carbohydrates doesn't overtax the body and send it into overdrive the way refined or processed sugars do.

Pasta is also a complex carbohydrate. The problem with pasta is that it is a "contrived" food. It has been processed, cooked, and mangled into a "near-food." There aren't enough vitamins, minerals, and enzymes in processed foods such as pasta to digest them. If you eat a lot of pasta, your body will have to take the necessary enzymes and other digestive aids from other areas of the body. Eventually, the supply of helpers will run out. The more extensively food is processed, the fewer natural nutrients are available for other uses. For example, enzymes in food help to digest food in the stomach. If the enzymes are destroyed in processing, they can't do their job in the stomach.

Carbohydrates that are "unavailable" to your body are those that humans can't digest: cellulose in vegetables, fruits, and grains. But these carbohydrates are important to health, because they constitute the fiber that adds bulk to help keep the bowels in good working order. Also, excess dietary fats that could contribute to high serum cholesterol are helped on their way out of the body by the roughage of fiber. The old adage, "An apple a day keeps the doctor away," was based on the need to keep the elimination system in shape. Today, oat bran is the "fiber of choice." Oat bran and other fiber-laden foods are now touted as the "magic cure" for keeping your arteries free of plaque. Of course, when the apple saying came about, folks were eating fewer refined food products to clog arteries. You can get a better cleansing effect from high fiber fruits, vegetables, and whole grains or rice than you get from so-called fiber-enriched processed foods. Refined carbohydrates lacking in fiber create havoc with your arteries and health. The more food is processed, the less fiber it contains.

FATS

Although we think of fats as being exclusive to the animal world, we also get fats from plants.

Fats are stored energy. There's more energy packed into a gram of fat than there is in a gram of either carbohydrate or protein. "Average Americans receive approximately 15 percent of their energy from protein, about 40 percent from fat, and 45 percent from carbohydrates"[7] Compare these figures with those of other populations, such as the people in Mongolia, who receive about 85 percent of their energy from carbohydrates.

Carbohydrates and proteins in foods are in a watery mix. Consequently, the proportion of carbohydrates or protein in a food is only
about 25 per cent of the weight of the food. Not so with fats. They
don't mix with water. Fats are fats 100 percent.

More oxygen is needed to metabolize fats than to metabolize
either protein or carbohydrates. It takes 100 molecules of oxygen to
form 70 molecules of carbon dioxide from fat. With protein oxidation you get 80 molecules of carbon dioxide from the same 100
molecules of oxygen, and carbohydrates give you a one-to-one return.[8] More fat in your diet means that more oxygen must be used to
metabolize it, and more acid produced; therein lies the rub. Fat in
and of itself isn't the big problem in American's arteries and health;
its the acid produced by fat metabolism and the acid from the foods
the fat is contained in that causes problems.

Americans are on a fight-food-fat crusade. The principal concern
about dietary fat is that it contributes to the cholesterol level, clogs arteries, and in turn, restricts or shuts down the supply of blood to the
heart. While that may be a valid reason for cutting down on the
amount of fatty meats you eat, it isn't the whole picture. Remember,
your body produces about sixty percent of your cholesterol. The bad
news about fats, an even greater concern than cholesterol, is that fats
are acid producers. Although they leave a neutral ash, metabolism of
the fats generates acid, and when fats are accompanied by meat even
more internal acid is generated.

The good news about fat is that, like sugar, the metabolic acid
can be eliminated through the lungs rather than through the kidneys. When your body must handle excessive amounts of acid, your
physiological processes run into trouble. As long as you can keep
breathing, you can eliminate acid from fats through the lungs.
When the acid level of your system gets too high from too much
protein, it is a whole-body condition. No matter how fast you pant,
breathing won't get rid of acid that must be eliminated through the
kidneys.

Most fat gets into your digestive system as a close companion of
animal protein. After a prolonged continuous diet of meats, the pH
of the body drops, and any additional acid may be enough to spark a
heart attack, especially if you exercise strenuously after eating. Your
vital organs must operate in a slightly alkaline environment. Too
much dietary fat is one situation that upsets the balance. Urine and

saliva pH tests can show you if your pH scales have tipped to the acid side.

ENZYMES

There are hundreds of different enzymes. Enzymes are protein substances produced by living cells. We produce enzymes and we ingest enzymes with our food. Some enzymes move nutrients through the digestive tract into the body; others act throughout the body as catalysts for different metabolic functions. Enzymes are the substances that allow the body to perform complicated chemical reactions at room temperature.

Enzymes from food provide the vitality the body needs to carry on life. Without a non-stop adequate supply of enzymes from raw, whole, living foods, the body can't properly replenish and rebuild cells. Enzymes, like just about everything else, do their best work in a favorable environment.

WELLNESS PRINCIPLE: *Enzymes are the key to all life.*

Enzymes are produced by living plants and animals. They cause changes in other substances without being changed themselves. In living plants, enzymes serve a metabolic function of building new tissue. However, they can be destroyed by cooking and be rendered inert by refrigeration. If fruit is refrigerated after it is picked, it won't ripen properly. Enzymes are ripening agents but cold temperatures keep them from working.

At some time you have probably bought a beautiful, succulent-looking peach from the cooled produce section of the supermarket. You bit into the magnificent specimen of nature in eager anticipation of savoring a ripe, sweet, juicy treat. Instead, your senses were startled by a hard, bitter impostor. The fruit had been picked and shipped to the store before it was ripe. Although the color was good, the maturing process had not been completed. Had you put your prize peach on the window sill for a couple of days, the enzymes would have again performed their magic and you would have had a succulent, mature piece of fruit instead of a ripe-retarded look-alike.

The enzymes in whole food act to complete the food's development and maturing. If the ripening process isn't interrupted by heat or cold, it continues until the food disintegrates—it rots. Overripe fruit and rotten potatoes have a lot in common—non-stop enzymatic activity. When the same disintegrating process takes place inside the body, it's termed digestion. The function of enzymes in fruits or vegetables doesn't change just because they are in the stomach. These enzymes can continue to work in an acid environment; enzymes from the pancreas can't.

Meat is affected by enzymes also. Seldom is an animal butchered and the meat immediately tossed onto the stove. Muscles harden soon after an animal is slaughtered; rigor mortis sets in. Stiffening develops as the pH drops and the muscle becomes more acid. The muscle hardens as it loses its capacity to retain water. If the meat has hung for a few days and the enzymes in the meat have a chance to work, water is again retained and the muscles soften. In essence, they begin to self destruct. Then they are ripe for eating.

Prime beef is sometimes allowed to hang in a refrigerator for up to ten days or two weeks. Green mold forms on it. Then it's "prime," "aged." It is deteriorated beef, tender, but rotting with the aid of enzymes.

Enzymes in saliva begin to ready food in the mouth for digestion. Enzymes also help to begin the digestive process in the stomach. When we eat whole food, living enzymes in that food initiate the digestion of the food that carried it in. Raw fruits and vegetables contain all of the enzymes necessary to almost completely digest their constituent parts: carbohydrates, proteins, and fats.

Those portions of carbohydrates, proteins, and fats that aren't completely digested by their own enzymes pass into the duodenum. The chemical structure of the substance and the enzymes of the pancreas continue the job of digesting the food. Pancreatic enzymes act as a backup, or finishing touch, to the natural digestion initiated by the enzymes in the food.

Enzymatic action in seeds and grains can be put on "hold" by enzyme inhibitors. You may have heard of archaeologists unearthing grains and seeds that had been entombed for hundreds of years. Grains and seeds are living entities that can lie dormant for long periods, then germinate when moisture and temperature conditions are right. Until conditions are favorable, enzyme inhibitors in seeds postpone the initiation of enzymatic action that begins the sprouting process. Warm temperatures and moist conditions override enzyme inhibitors and allow the enzymes to go to work. Enzyme inhibitors can be deactivated either by sprouting or by cooking.

Cooking dormant seeds and grains destroys the enzyme inhibitors but it also destroys enzymes. Under conditions that allow seeds or grains to germinate, enzymes are released to inhibit the inhibitors.

Enzyme inhibitors cause digestive distress if seeds and grains are eaten while the inhibitors have the upper hand. This is why soy protein is so hard to digest; it has the highest known concentration of enzyme inhibitors.

The pattern of enzymatic activity of food crops can be influenced by farming methods. Modern agricultural practices allow for faster, more extensive and efficient methods of collecting crops from fields. In the past, grain remained on the stalk in the field after cutting. During this time the grain was exposed to moisture and sunlight, which allowed enzymes to be released and produced, and the germination process to begin. Grains are now removed from the stalk immediately after cutting. This practice is more economical than former methods, but a vital transition period is eliminated.

Current practices deliver mature but dormant grains to food processors to be transformed into virtually enzyme-free products. Enzymes may be added to consumer products artificially. This practice is helpful in the manufacturing of bread and bakery products, but the added enzymes are of little or no benefit to the person who eats the food. Man cannot improve on the nutritional value of food that is grown in naturally rich soil.

WELLNESS PRINCIPLE: *Mother Nature prepares the best food, and it's your choice how you eat it.*

CALCULATING PROTEIN CONSUMPTION

The list of foods that follows is not all-inclusive by any means. It is intended merely to serve as a guide for estimating how much protein you get when you eat some common (and perhaps not so com-

mon) foods of the average American's daily fare. The amount of protein ascribed to each food is a rough, but close, approximation. It
makes very little difference to your body whether you are consuming
120 grams or protein a day or 113 grams—it's still too much.

By using these figures, you will have a good idea of the amount of
protein you are asking your body to contend with each day. However, the purpose is to help you be *aware* of how much protein you
are eating, not to turn you into a gram-counting fanatic. Just remember that meat, eggs, and dairy products aren't the only sources of
protein. Almost all food contains protein!

I don't recommend all of the foods shown on this list. The list is
to give you an idea of the foods that are the most acid-producing for
your body.

PROTEIN CONTENT OF SOME COMMON FOODS*

	Quantity	Protein in grams
Almonds	13	2.4
Apples	1	.2
Apricots, raw	1/2 cup	1
, dried	1/2 cup	3.5
Asparagus, cut from frozen	1 cup	6
Avocados	1/2	2
Bacon	2 slices	4
Bagels, egg (3" diam.)	1	6
Bananas	1	1
Barley	1/2 cup	8
Beans, dried (Great Northern)	1 cup	14
, dried, (Navy)	1 cup	15
, canned, Red Kidney	1 cup	15
Beans, green	1 cup	2
Beef, steak (sirloin) broiled	3 oz	20
, ground, 10% fat, broiled	3 oz	23
, roast, lean and fat	3 oz	17
Beet greens	1 cup	2
Beets	1 cup	2
Blackberries	1 cup	2
Blueberries	1 cup	1

PROTEIN CONTENT OF SOME COMMON FOODS*
(Cont'd)

	Quantity	Protein in grams
Bran flakes (40% bran) w/sugar	1 cup	4
Bran, oat	2 oz	10.3
Bran, wheat	3.5 oz	12
Brazil nuts	1 oz	4
Bread, white	1 slice	2
Bread, whole wheat	1 slice	3
Broccoli	1 cup	5
Brussels sprouts (frozen)	1 cup	5
Butter	1 oz	.2
Cabbage	1 cup	1
Cantaloupe	1/2 melon	2
Carob flour	1/2 cup	2.38
Carrots	1 cup	1
Cashew nuts, roasted in oil	1/2 cup	12
Cauliflower	1 cup	3
Celery	1 cup	1
Chard	3.5 oz	1.4
Cheese, cheddar	1 oz	7
, cottage, lg. curd	1/2 cup	14
, cream	1 oz	2
Cherries, sour	1 cup	2
, sweet	10	1
Chicken, breast, boneless	2.8 oz	26
, drumstick, boneless	1.3 oz	12
Codfish, broiled	3.5 oz	28.5
Cornflakes	1 cup	2
Corn, frozen kernels	1 cup	1
, on the cob (5" ear)	1	4
Corn oil		-0-
Corn Syrup		-0-
Corned beef, canned	3 oz	22
, hash	1 cup	19
Crab meat, canned	1 cup	24
Crackers, rye, whole grain	2 wafers	2
, soda	4 (one packet)	1
Cranberry sauce	1/2 cup	.1

PROTEIN CONTENT OF SOME COMMON FOODS*
(Cont'd)

	Quantity	Protein in grams
Cucumbers (not pared)	3.5 oz	.9
Dates, whole	10	2
, chopped	1 cup	4
Donuts, cake type	1	1
, yeast	1	3
Eggs	1	6
Figs, dried	4 oz.	3.5
Flour, white (all purpose)	1 cup	1
Flour, whole wheat	1 cup	2
Grapefruit	1/2	1
, juice, frozen	1 cup	1
Grapes, white seedless	5.64 oz	1.6
Haddock, fried, breaded	3 oz	17
Honey		-0-
Honeydew melon	3.5 oz	.8
Hot Dog	1	6
Ice cream, regular	3-fl oz	2
, soft-serve	1 cup	7
Kale, frozen	1 cup	4
Lamb, chop, lean and fat	3.1 oz	18
, leg, roasted	3 oz	22
Lemons	1	1
Lentils, whole, cooked	1 cup	16
Lettuce, iceberg	1/4 head	1
, romaine (chopped)	1 cup	1
Lima beans, dried	1 cup	16
, baby	1 cup	13
, Fordhook	1 cup	10
Lime juice	1 cup	1
Lobster	3.5 oz	18.7
Macaroni, cooked	1 cup	5 - 7
Milk, cow's, whole	1 cup	8
, nonfat	1 cup	8
Milk, goat's, whole	1 cup	8
Millet, cooked	1 cup	2.8

PROTEIN CONTENT OF SOME COMMON FOODS*
(Cont'd)

	Quantity	Protein in grams
Molasses		-0-
Mushrooms	1 cup	2
Oatmeal	1 cup	5
Okra	10 pods	2
Olive oil		-0-
Onions (chopped)	1 cup	3
Oranges	1	1
Orange juice (froz. con.)	1 cup	2
Oysters, raw	1 cup	20
Parsnips, diced	1 cup	2
Peaches, raw	1	1
, canned	1 cup	1
Peanut butter	1 tbsp	4
Peanuts	1/2 cup	18.5
Pears	1	1
Peas, dried split	1 cup	16
Peas, green (frozen)	1 cup	8
Pike, Northern, raw	4 oz	21.9
Pineapple, raw, diced	1 cup	1
, juice, canned	1 cup	1
Pizza, cheese (12" diam.)	1/8 sec.	6
Plums, canned	3	1
Pork, chop (lean and fat)	2.7 oz	19
, roast (lean only)	2.4 oz	20
Potato salad w/cooked dressing	1 cup	7
Potatoes, french fries	10 (2 - 3 1/2")	2
, hashed brown frozen	1 cup	3
, sweet (baked)	1 (5"x2")	2
, white (baked)	1/2 lb	4
Prunes, dried	5 large	1
Radishes	3.5 oz	1
Raisins (loose packed)	1 cup	4
Raspberries, raw, whole	1 cup	1
Refined sugar		-0-
Rhubarb, sugar added	1 cup	1

PROTEIN CONTENT OF SOME COMMON FOODS*
(Cont'd)

	Quantity	Protein in grams
Rice, brown, cooked	1 cup	4.88
Rice, white, cooked	1 cup	4.10
Salmon, canned	3 oz	17
Sardines, canned in oil	3 oz	20
Sauerkraut, canned	1 cup	2
Sausage, brown and serve	1 link	3
Scallops, frozen, breaded	6	16
, steamed	3.5 oz	23.2
Shrimp, fried	3.5 oz	20.3
, canned	3 oz	21
Soy beans, cooked from dry	1 cup	28.6
Spaghetti, "al dente"	1 cup	7
, tender	1 cup	5
, canned, w/tom sauce & cheese	1 cup	6
, canned, w/tom sauce & mtballs	1 cup	12
Spinach, raw (chopped)	1 cup	2
, frozen (chopped)	1 cup	6
Squash, summer	1 cup	2
, winter (baked)	1 cup	4
Strawberries	1 cup	1
Sunflower seeds	3.5 oz	24
Tangerines	1	1
Tomatoes, raw (2 3/5" diam.)	1	1
, canned	1 cup	2
, juice (canned)	6 oz	2
Tuna	3.5 oz	28
Turkey	3.5 oz	27
Turnips	1 cup	1
Turnip Greens (froz. chopped)	1 cup	4
Veal, cutlet, braised/broiled	3 oz	23
Vegetables, frozen mixed	1 cup	6
Walnuts, black, chopped	1 cup	26
, English, chopped	1 cup	18
Watercress	3.5 oz	2.2
Watermelon	4" x 8" wedge w/rind	2

PROTEIN CONTENT OF SOME COMMON FOODS*
(Cont'd)

	Quantity	Protein in grams
Wheat germ	1 tbsp	2
Yogurt, plain	8 oz	12

*The protein content figures are based on information from several sources. ([1] "Food Processor II." [2] Guthrie, Helen A., Ph.D., D.Sc., R.D., *Introductory Nutrition*, Fifth Edition. St. Louis, Toronto, London: The C.V. Mosby Company, 1983, pp. 608 -641.[3] Robinson, Corinne H., *Proudfit-Robinson's Normal and Therapeutic Nutrition*, 13th Edition. New York: The Macmillan Company, 1967, pp. 764 - 806. [4] Thomas, Clayton L., M.D., M.P.H., ed., *Taber's Cyclopedic Medical Dictionary*. Philadelphia, F. A. David Company, 1985, pp. 2060 - 2075.)

CHAPTER 21

Funny Foods and Phoney Foods

There's nothing man can do to improve the nutritional quality of food grown by nature. Man's alleged improvements can only enhance flavor (to suit his well-conditioned tastes), prolong shelf life, and add commercial appeal. Despite claims of "new and improved," "fortified," or "vitamin enriched," processed foods lack the health-giving vitality of whole foods. Refined, enriched white bread typifies the technological degradation of a wholesome food. A large portion of the highly nutritious ingredients inherent in whole wheat flour is refined away to produce a more profitable, less nutritious product.

Nutrients may be replaced in refined foods, but the replacements are made to man's specifications. Man's conscious mind determines the kinds, ratios, and formulae of ingredients that go into refined foods. The end results may or may not conform to nature's specifications. White flour, an end product of a refining process, makes more delicate cakes and finer breads than wheat flour. However, nutritional benefits are sacrificed on the altar of convenience, appearance, and cultivated tastes. The violence done in refining whole wheat flour into white flour is an excellent example of man's philosophy: "If it can be done, it should be done"—especially if it's profitable.

The figures in the table below were taken from a graph pub-lished in the 1977 Dietary Goals of the United States. It's obvious that refining and processing considerably reduces the nutritive value of whole wheat; and this is just one example of how we van-dalize nature's craftwork.

VITAMINS AND MINERALS LOST IN REFINING WHOLE WHEAT
(Adapted from "Dietary Goals for the United States," U.S. Government Printing Office, Washington: 1977)

NUTRIENTS THAT MAY BE LOST IN REFINING WHOLE WHEAT

	Potential Loss %
Vitamin B_1 (thiamin)	90
Vitamin B_2 (riboflavin)	70
Vitamin B_3 (niacin, nicotinic acid)	70
Vitamin B_6 (pyrodoxine)	80
Pantothenic Acid	50
Folic Acid	70
Biotin	80
Vitamin E	50
Calcium	50
Iron	80
Copper	60
Magnesium	70
Potassium	50
Zinc	70

These startling figures show the potential loss of nutrients through the refining of only one staple of life. Hundreds of "phony" foods that have suffered equal or more severe nutritional dismemberment are touted on TV and stocked on supermarket shelves.

WELLNESS PRINCIPLE: *The best thing to be said about eating foods promoted in TV advertisements is: "Don't!"*

HEALTH INHIBITORS

Processed foods and refined foods are "phony" foods that inhibit health. They are foreign to your body even if you have been consuming them for years. They are strangers that excite your body to adapt its natural way of functioning. Physiological adaptation leads to disease and discomfort.

Margarine is one of the most common phony foods in use today. Margarine may be made from vegetable oils, but these oils have been mutilated. Margarine is hydrogenated in processing. Additional hydrogen ions are added to the vegetable oils. Margarine is one of the worst processed foods you can put in your body.

The adaptations your body must make to process inappropriate food can be compared with the concessions it makes to other unusual circumstances. For instance, if you walk around with an unnecessary lift in one shoe, or in shoes with different height heels, your body can adapt to the unnatural situation. However, after a while, you'll experience aches and pains in your legs, back, and other areas of your body that are even farther removed from your feet. Although the connection between the symptom and the cause may not be obvious, it is direct. Phony foods act in much the same way. If you don't understand the universal effect food has on your body, it may not be apparent that your diet is the source of your physical distress; but the distress itself is obvious.

Phony foods are health inhibitors. Some, like salt and spices, although grown in or mined from the ground, are useless to your body because they contain elements that provide no nutrition. Others, like soft drinks and processed meats, are detrimental to your body because they contain substances with few natural enzymes, overstimulate the body, and waste the minerals of the alkaline reserve. They inhibit natural healthful healing and replenishing because the body must adapt its natural functions to accommodate the highly-processed, industrial-strength foods.

Your body's ability to adapt to health-inhibiting foods is a survival technique. This talent for adaptation should be called on only in emergencies, not two or three times a day. The goal of eating—if you want to be and stay healthy—is to give your body the whole foods it was designed to process, foods that provide fuel for generating energy and replenishing cells.

Vegetables that have been irradiated for cosmetic purposes, as mentioned in Chapter 10, may be appealing to the eye; however, the effects of eating irradiated foods have yet to be documented. Companies that use this process don't even tell us about it. What does irradiation do to the natural bonding of food? Does it "kill" the natural bonding of food just as surely as it kills the bacteria?

I am not suggesting that the residual radiation level is harmful. But I am questioning the wisdom of tampering with the only source of live food in our markets. The body can adapt its function to handle "deformed" foods for a time before it becomes exhausted. Heaping irradiated substances on top of other processed foods may contribute to the body becoming exhausted faster.

You can help to protect yourself against unknowingly buying irradiated vegetables and fruits by asking your grocer to sign a statement that the produce you buy from his store has not been irradiated. If he resists endorsing his produce, you can assume that it has, indeed, been irradiated.

Equally as important as providing body-ready foods is protecting your body from substances that masquerade as food but counteract health because they are either useless or toxic. Many of the foods that are staples of our daily diets stimulate the body. If you consume many of the foods included in the following list, your body is being run by external stimulation. If you can't go more than two hours without being jacked up with one of the substances on this list, you are being controlled by external stimulants. Your body's ability to regulate itself has been overridden by a constant tide of stimulants. When the effect of the stimulants has run its course, you feel "hungry" again. By slowly progressing from health-inhibiting foods to health-inducing foods your body gains control of its own operations and lets you know when it is time to refuel. A person who is truly healthy can eat a meal and not be hungry or "unsatisfied" for at least four hours.

COMMON HEALTH INHIBITORS
AND EXTERNAL PHYSIOLOGY REGULATORS

Stimulants	Condiments	Altered Foods
Drugs	Salt	Fried Foods
Coffee	Herb Teas	Margarine
Tea	Spices	Pasteurized Milk
Carbonated Beverages		Ice Cream
Alcohol		
Tobacco		

Processed Foods	Refined Foods
Processed Meats	White Sugar
Ham	White Flour
Bacon	Pies, Cookies, Cakes
Hot Dogs	Macaroni
Salami	Spaghetti
Bologna	Crackers

EXPANSIVE AND CONTRACTIVE FOODS

Expansive and contractive foods are "funny" foods. They do strange things to your attitudes and your body.

Everything you eat causes a physiological response. Physiological responses to foods can affect the way you feel; they can affect your attitude and personality; and, most importantly, they can damage your health. Some common, every-day foods like eggs or dairy products cause digestive upsets in some people; sugar can make others hyperactive, and processed foods can devitalize your systems. Different foods can have different effects.

Most foods can be classified as either *expansive* or *contractive*. As a general rule, alkalizing foods can be considered expansive, and acidifying foods contractive.

Expansive "foods" like drugs, alcohol, sugar, and coffee can be temporarily stimulating. Expansive foods are processed quickly and have an expansive effect. (Recall the "mind expanding" description of some recreational drugs.) The body's metabolic rate picks up for a short period. Even fruit juices have a slightly expansive effect. You can drink too much fruit juice. A good gauge for determining how much is too much is to consider how much is in one unit of the fruit and not drink more juice than you would get in the number of units you can eat. For example, if you can eat three oranges, the amount of juice you should drink is the amount you would get in three oranges.

The combination of sugar and fruit juice is especially likely to produce coughing. Many children get this combination almost daily in some prepared "fruit" drinks.

Consuming large quantities of fruit juice when you have a cold may stimulate coughing due to the expansive effect of the fruit juice. Since a cold is a cleansing process and expansive fruit juice can increase coughing, you can see why the traditional contractive chicken soup treatment for a cold makes you feel better.

After eating expansive foods, we (or our cells) are stimulated to function faster. We feel, to a greater or lesser degree, that we can run faster and jump higher, solve the problems of the world, drive just a little farther or faster, or cope with the job a little while longer. We are stimulated.

> **WELLNESS PRINCIPLE:** *Expansive substances are often used as a crutch to help us limp through life.*

Contractive foods, on the other hand, have the opposite effect on the body. Foods such as meat and salt have a restricting effect on blood vessels, cells, and even thinking. Butter, which seems innocuous enough, has a slightly contractive effect. Energy is focused on taking care of internal matters. The body "draws in," or contracts its resources inward. The body must devote a lot of attention to processing contractive foods. Energies are directed toward metabolizing usable parts of contractive food, storing surpluses, and casting out unusable materials.

Between expansive and contractive lie the neutral foods: fruits, vegetables, grains, nuts, seeds, and beans. Fruits and vegetables are essentially neutral but they lean toward the expansive side. Grains and beans are essentially neutral but teeter toward the contractive side.

The following diagram illustrates some common expansive and contractive foods.

EXPANSIVE	NEUTRAL FOODS		CONTRACTIVE
Drugs			
Liquor			
Beer			Salt
Wine			Red Meat
Sugar			Fowl
Syrup(Honey, Molasses)			Eggs
Chocolate		Beans	Fish
Coffee		Seeds	Chicken
Tea	Fruits	Nuts	Cheese
Fruit Juice	Vegetables	Grains	Butter

Expansive and contractive foods are stressful to the body. However, the body is a balance-seeking mechanism. If you consume a lot of one highly expansive substance (like alcohol), you'll crave a contractive substance (like salt) to balance it. You can see why margaritas are so popular—alcohol and salt all in one package. Beer and pretzels, wine and cheese, and coffee following a meal are standard combinations that perform balancing acts.

Your body constantly works to maintain balance. If you give it contractive foods only, it *will* balance the restrictive effect. Energy that has been directed inward will rebound outward. The balancing process may take the form of explosive outbursts of temper. Volatile behavior is a personality trait that can develop from a diet made up predominantly of contractive foods.

Similarly, a strict vegetarian who eats only expansive fruits and vegetables may develop food-induced personality quirks. A strict vegetarian may have fruit juice for breakfast, carrot juice for lunch, and a salad for dinner. With no contractive foods as balancing agents, he may become so "spaced out" he is unable to concentrate. One thought tumbles on top of another, or his mind wanders and he isn't able to carry a thought through to completion. Internal activity is balanced by a "laid back," "mellow" exterior.

In the same vein, the effect sugar has on some children and some adults is a symptom of physiological balance-seeking. Many youngsters stigmatized with the "hyperactive" label have been found to settle down to normal levels of activity when expansive sugar is restricted from their diets. Balance is the key to a healthy body, a healthy attitude, and a healthy personality.

There is another wrinkle associated with imbalances brought about by expansive and contractive foods—cravings.

Diets tipped dramatically to either the expansive or contractive side bring about food cravings. Eliminating a contractive food from your diet without eliminating an expansive food can generate a craving for the balancing agent. Cravings can be strong enough to weaken even the most sincere resolution to improve eating habits.

You probably eat enough of a variety of foods to have favorites in both expansive and contractive categories; very likely you are reasonably well-balanced. However, when you commit to improving your health and decide to eliminate a particular food such as coffee from the expansive side, you should also eliminate a counterbalancing frequently eaten food such as eggs from the contractive side. Keep the two sides equally weighted. Imagine a group of children of comparable weight on a see-saw, four on one end and four on the other. If Johnny jumps off one end, Jimmy had better abandon ship on the other, or the see-saw will be out of balance and won't work the way it was designed.

WELLNESS PRINCIPLE: *Food affects your personality as well as your health.*

COOKED FOOD

Cooking demolishes the quality of rawness that we will talk about in the next chapter. Anything that has been heated above 120°F has been cooked. Cooking strengthens the bonds of food elements and destroys enzymes. The stomach is where food is prepared to be digested. It is supposed to act as a receptacle for food that contains enzymes. Food that has been cooked can't contribute the enzymes necessary to begin the digestive process.

Enzymes act as a catalyst to get digestion going. Without enzymes, the digestive process is hampered. As a result, pancreatic enzymes are left with the burden of breaking down food particles. The pancreas is supposed to be the clean-up brigade, not the full force.

Your body can handle cooked foods and gain nutrients from them. However, your systems don't get the benefit from cooked foods that they get from raw foods. Consequently, metabolic efficiency is reduced. Inefficiency in any system of the body adds unnecessary stress to the whole body.

SUPPLEMENTS

"New," wonder nutrients periodically come into vogue as the latest panacea for heart disease, cancer, or general aging. Vitamins C and E held the limelight about twenty years ago. Lecithin hit the big time soon after that. Now, as we race headlong into the last decade of the twentieth century, oat bran is touted as the answer to our health prayers. Surely, as a nation, we will soon recognize that you can't treat bits and pieces of the body and expect to get whole-body health. Even a nationally known pharmaceutical company (Hoffmann-La Roche, Inc.) acknowledged in a full-page magazine advertisement that supplements are "not substitutes for a variety of good foods."

WELLNESS PRINCIPLE: *Health comes from inside out.*

Supplements are also "funny foods." They are food that the body may be able to use, but most supplements are either inorganic or incomplete. Some supplements, like enzymes, are parts of real food; others, like dolomite, are inorganic minerals that may fool the body into treating them like usable substances for a while, but end up being deposited where they aren't needed. Eventually, they may even cause problems.

Most people who take vitamin and mineral supplements believe they are solving a particular problem. They are trying to find the magic formula that will add energy, build bones, calm nerves, slow aging, or give them some other specific benefit. Unfortunately, supplements don't make you healthy. You may feel better for a while because of the added stimulation to the body; but supplements may not *correct the cause* of your concern even if they make you feel better.

A patient came to me complaining of allergies. She had with her a grocery bag full of vitamin and mineral supplements for my assessment. She claimed she was essentially in excellent health and attributed her vigor to a vast array of nutrition supplements.

As we talked, she enumerated how many tablets, grams, or International Units she took of each, and what they did for her. She was one of the most knowledgeable supplement-takers I have ever encountered.

Four years earlier, the lady told me, she had been feeling tired, so she started taking vitamin B. Later she added vitamin C, then iron. As time went by, she added more and more vitamins and minerals. I don't know the exact number of different pills she was taking when I met her, but it was impressive.

"Now," she told me, "if I don't take my supplements, I feel worse than I did before I started."

"I'm confused," I told her after she had finished her travelogue through Vitamin Land. "You said that you started out taking one or two vitamin Bs and Cs and added a little iron. Now you're taking more vitamin B, more vitamin C and iron, and all of these other things as well."

"That's right. And I feel *great*—as long as I take them."

Try as I might, I had trouble understanding her logic.

"That sounds backwards," I observed. "I can understand that four years ago when your lifestyle and diet were terrible and you were sick, you might have needed a grocery bag full of supplements temporarily. But if the supplements were making you better, you should have been down to half a grocery bag full after two years and taking maybe one or two specific supplements after four years. It seems to me that your supplement program isn't correcting your problem and may be contributing to it." The allergic reactions she had come to me about were a signal that her body had to devote much of its energy to taking care of the flood of strange nutrients.

When we take supplements, we are getting isolated elements that we should be getting from whole foods. It's rather like taking statements out of context; you might get full benefit, but more than likely what you get is distorted.

Picking and choosing the elements you think your body needs is chancy at best. We are designed to operate as a whole entity. Parts of foods don't supply enzymes and other collateral substances that help your body to process the parts. You can actually take enough supplements of individual nutrients to cause symptoms of a deficiency of that or other nutrients.

I'm not saying that we never need supplements. Occasionally, we may need supplementation to give a boost to our digestive and assimilative processes so that we can extract and use all of the nutrients available in whole foods. When we take supplements to "treat" a specific condition, we are focusing on a symptom rather than the problem. We *need* whole foods that contain all of the ingredients necessary for our bodies to function properly.

If supplements are required for short-term therapy, they should be organic—made from plants. Supplements that are made of inorganic materials aren't as suitable for human metabolism as those from organic sources. Our bodies were not designed to break the powerful ionic bonds that connect substances of the mineral kingdom.

Calcium supplements, for instance, may deposit calcium in your body, but not necessarily in your bones or teeth. Dolomite is calcium magnesium carbonate. It comes from limestone. Dolomite hasn't been processed through either the plant or animal kingdoms. Consequently, its ingredients haven't been converted to a form we can use.

There is, however, a form of calcium supplementation that your body can use: Lemon Egg (sometimes called egg calcium). Lemon Egg is an easily made home brew containing all natural ingredients: freshly squeezed lemon juice and fresh, clean, uncooked whole eggs. Your body can take the calcium from Lemon Egg and put it to work where it is needed. It also has the added alkaline ash benefits inherent in fresh lemon juice; it contributes alkaline properties to your body along with the calcium. Although Lemon Egg isn't cooked to "kill the germs," most bacteria, including salmonella, cannot survive the acid environment of lemon juice. First, how to concoct it:

LEMON EGG
The Ultimate in Calcium Supplementation

Carefully place whole, clean, uncooked, uncracked eggs in a clean wide-mouth jar. Cover the eggs with *freshly squeezed* lemon juice. (Concentrated lemon juice is not a substitute—it has been pasteurized.) Cover the jar loosely and place it in the refrigerator. A few times during the day, gently—very gently —agitate the liquid in the jar. As the calcium from the shells is leached by the lemon juice, bubbles will appear around the eggs.

After approximately 48 hours, when the bubbling has stopped, carefully remove the eggs from the jar. Be sure not to break the egg membrane.

Replace the lid tightly on the jar containing the liquid and shake the mixture. *Voila!* Lemon Egg.

You will notice when you remove the eggs from the liquid that the "shells" are soft. The citric acid from the lemon juice has combined with calcium from the egg shells to form calcium citrate. This calcium is organic in nature and usable by your body; it comes from plant and animal sources. It retains its living quality.

After the calcium has been leached from the shells, the eggs can be used in the same way you would normally use uncooked eggs. If you leave the eggs in the mixture for more than forty-eight hours, two things will happen: the mixture will begin to thicken, and the eggs will absorb more of the lemon flavor through the soft membrane.

Lemon Egg mixture is an excellent, high-powered, *short-term* calcium supplement. One-half teaspoonful each day will give you all of the additional calcium you need to begin to rebuild your calcium supply. Like any supplement, this one will give your body resources with which to work while more covalent calcium laden foods are being introduced into your diet. Green leafy vegetables such as kale, watercress, mustard greens and turnip greens are vegetable sources of calcium.

The amount of Lemon Egg you take is important. Taking too much can induce symptoms you won't like. One-half teaspoonful is all of the Lemon Egg you need *each day* for thirty days. Taking more than one-half teaspoonful a day can lead to leg cramps, the same symptom that is associated with too little calcium.

Supplements can be helpful on a short-term basis. I'm not anti-supplements. They should be the kind that help your body get the vitamins and minerals from the food you eat rather than attempt to supply the vitamins and minerals that are missing. Supplements serve a useful purpose when taken only occasionally, as needed. Your goal is to give your body all of the nutrients it needs in the form it can use. You don't need to add fragments of food to round out a proper diet. When you eat the foods you were designed to eat, you will have a hard time not being healthy.

As we become sicker, we try to regulate our bodies from the outside by diet and medications: vitamins, minerals, antacids, diuretics, anti-inflammatories, and on and on. Given the opportunity and the right environment, the body can regulate itself internally. When you keep your personal castle balanced, synchronized, and properly fueled, good health is inevitable.

CHAPTER 22

More About Foods

Selecting foods for everyday eating needn't become an obsession. You already have an eating lifestyle that you developed without much conscious effort. You can modify the way you eat without completely disrupting your life. All you need is (1) the desire to be healthier, and (2) awareness of the effects of substances you ask your body to process. Gradual modification is the key to developing a healthy eating lifestyle. Give the internal you as much consideration as you give the external. As you embark on your journey to life-long health, become more aware of the foods you are now eating by evaluating their qualities.

QUALITIES OF FOOD

You can evaluate foods by their qualities. Five essential qualities are inherent in "good" foods. The more of these qualities a given food can claim, the better that food is for you. To rate a nutritional 5-star quality award, a food should be:

1. Whole
2. Raw
3. Alkaline ash-producing
4. Satisfying in moderate quantities
5. Compatible with the human organism.

215

Wholeness

A good food retains its natural qualities, being as close to its natural state as possible. Fresh vegetables and fruits are nature's handiwork. They are whole and wholesome. Quick-frozen vegetables are second in line of desirability if fresh aren't available. Canned vegetables have been cooked and salted, but they are better than highly processed foods.

Whole wheat flour has also been processed. However, it is structurally closer to wheat as it comes from the field than is white flour.

A test question for wholeness: Is this food the same now as nature prepared it? If the answer is "Yes," the food is probably whole. If the answer is "No," the food has probably been corrupted and is no longer whole.

Rawness

Raw foods, plant and animal alike, retain more vitality than cooked or processed foods. The many elements that make up raw food are readily available to your body. In addition, raw foods carry with them enzymes that begin the digestive process. Of course, this is not an endorsement of eating raw meat, since meat is rarely fresh enough to be free of virulent elements that can make us sick.

Cooking destroys most of the noxious bacteria in meat. Cooking also destroys enzymes and alters bonds of vegetables. The bonds of cooked food aren't as strong as ionic bonds of the mineral kingdom, or as easily broken as covalent bonds. Recall the report cited in Chapter 16 of the cats that became sick and couldn't reproduce after they had been fed nothing but cooked food. Loosely connected covalent bonds are found naturally in the plant and animal kingdoms. Members of the animal kingdom are designed to eat covalently bonded foods. Their digestive systems work best on substances with bonds that are loosely held together and easily broken.

Many of us have lived on cooked, processed, and pickled foods for so long that our bodies are no longer accustomed to handling raw foods. We are functioning in a condition of physiological adaptation. We can sustain this pattern for years, but our health goes steadily downhill in the process.

If you are not accustomed to raw foods, reintroduce (or introduce) them into your diet slowly. Allow your body to re-tune gradually. Ideally, about thirty percent of your diet should consist of raw fruits and vegetables.

Ash

The ash quality of food is very important to long-term health. Seventy-five percent of the food we eat should leave an alkaline ash. The other twenty-five percent can be acid ash foods. The best acid ash foods are whole foods: grains, cereals, nuts, and seeds.

Physiological pH should lean slightly to the alkaline side of neutral. If we eat a lot of food that leaves an acid ash, our bodies will become acid. Too much phosphorus, too much sulfur, and too many nitrates consumed in food leads to a state of acidosis. If your body becomes highly acidotic, it can't function properly and ultimately will shut down.

Satiety

Non-stop eating may fill your stomach, but it won't necessarily completely satisfy your hunger. Hunger is satisfied when your body has the nutrients it needs. However, your body doesn't need to be saturated with vitamins and minerals. You need only enough for your body to be able to function as well as possible for as long as possible.

Your body can assimilate only a given amount of food. Every system in the body has its physiological limit. Quantity limitations control the amount of food the body can digest and assimilate. These limitations are imposed by factors including the overall state of health. When the limits are exceeded, natural digestion falters. Yet something must be done with all of the food that has been consumed. Even if it can't be assimilated, food will continue to decompose until it is eliminated. Unusable proteins, carbohydrates, and fats decompose in different ways:

Proteins putrefy	Gases generated by protein putrefaction cause "stomach rumblings," gas pains, and flatus odor.

Carbohydrates ferment   Fermentation also produces gas. Belching
                           can usually be associated with fermented
                           carbohydrates.

Fats rancidify   Fats are normally oxidized; however, if they
                           decompose only partially, the remainder can
                           become rancid

If you eat enough food to exceed the physiological limits of your
systems, the excess food will putrefy, ferment, or rancidify.

I believe the average American eats twice as much food as he
needs. If we took half of the food that's put on the average
American's meal table and sent it someplace else, two things would
happen: (1) We would be healthier, and (2) the people who ate it
would be sicker. In the first place, we consume more calories than we
need. In the second place, our food is so highly processed that it isn't
good for anyone even though we're used to it. We would be healthier
by reducing the amount of improper foods in our diets.

Your body tells you when you have supplied it with enough nutrition for the moment. In addition, your body tells you when it needs
to be refueled. There are two specific times you shouldn't eat: (1)
when you are not hungry, and (2) when your temperature is above
100°F.

We have a tendency to "eat by the clock": breakfast at 7:00, lunch
at noon, and dinner at 6:00 is a common schedule for many American families. However, ideally you should eat when your body tells
you it is time; not when the clock strikes.

And when you have a fever, your body is very busy cleaning out
and repairing itself. There is a solid basis for the old adage, "starve a
fever." You have probably noticed that when you have a fever, you
lose your appetite. Your body is telling you that it doesn't need
replenishing just then. So, don't eat until your temperature goes
down to under 100°F and your appetite returns. In the meantime,
drink only water—not fruit juice, just water.

You are much less likely to overeat good, whole foods than you
are to overeat processed, incomplete foods. Fragmented foods aren't
fully satisfying. Our bodies crave the parts that are missing. How

often do you leave the dinner table feeling full but not quite satisfied? It isn't that you haven't had enough to eat; it's that some essential nutrients are still missing. Often, sodium is the missing ingredient—not inorganic salt but organic sodium. You generally don't suffer from the I'm-full-but-I-want-something-else syndrome when you have had generous portions of vegetables with your meal. Your body knows when it has been satisfied.

Compatibility

A substance can be (1) whole, (2) raw, (3) alkaline ash-producing, and (4) satisfying in small quantities, yet lethal. The substances you consume must be classified as food, not poison. They must be compatible with the human organism. Most, but not all, poisonous substances we know about are man-made from plant derivatives. Foods must satisfy the *compatibility* qualification.

As a sample of the food-evaluation technique, we'll compare how apples, parsnips, and grains score on the Quality of Foods test.

An apple that comes straight from the tree

- is whole	1
- is raw	1
- leaves an alkaline ash	1
- satisfies the appetite	1
- is compatible with the human body.	1
A fresh apple scores	5

Parsnips, though, rack up a lower score. Parsnips are:

- whole food	1
- usually cooked, although they can be eaten raw	0
- alkaline ash-producing	1
- of a high satiety value—you're not likely to overeat parsnips	1
- compatible with the human body	1
Parsnips score	4

Grains can go either way, depending upon how you handle them.

Grains as they come from the fields are:

- whole food   1
- not suitable for consumption in raw form
    unless sprouted   0
- acid ash-producers   0
- satisfying   1
- compatible with our systems   1
                        Grains score only   3

However, if you sprout grain until it is about an inch long, it can be eaten raw. Sprouted grain leaves an alkaline ash. It scores a 5 for quality. You can take a 3-star grain, sprout it for use in salads, and turn it into a 5-star food.

FOOD COMBINING

Planning meals is an everyday occurrence for all of us. Even if the plan is merely selecting a restaurant where you will eat lunch—a seafood specialty, ethnic restaurant, haute cuisine, hamburger shop, or pizza parlor—you have a good idea of the foods available. For meals at home, we have our traditional favorites: combinations of foods we have enjoyed in the past, or the occasional venture into the unknown with new culinary creations. Selecting foods and combinations of foods is just part of living.

As science has learned more about how the body operates, we have come to understand that just dumping a motley assortment of food into our stomachs at a sitting isn't advantageous for us. Even good, wholesome foods lose some of their benefits when they are inappropriately combined with certain other foods.

A comprehensive review of the ins and outs of food-combining is beyond the scope of this book. However, other publications go into detail about which foods work together, and why. I will present here only a general overview of why it makes a difference how you combine foods at each meal.

In Elementary Eating 101, you learned that food goes from the mouth into the stomach. This is generally a rather orderly process. The manner in which food is stored in the stomach and processed out of the stomach is also orderly. It goes out in much the same sequence as it went in. A cup of coffee, a slice of cantaloup, and a bowl of corn flakes with sugar, raisins, and milk might all hit your stomach nearly simultaneously in the morning. That's as much as your consciousness must contend with in eating your morning meal. Next, it is up to your stomach to do something about sorting out the mess. The food must be broken down and prepared for digestion and assimilation.

Your internal intelligence knows exactly what pH is needed and how to handle each type of food that comes along. Carbohydrate, starch, and protein each require particular acid secretions and particular amounts of time for digestion. Proteins need a more acidic environment than carbohydrates. Carbohydrates and starches can be prepared for digestion much faster than protein. Your breakfast cantaloup and sugar, like other carbohydrates, ordinarily are digested very quickly—in about fifteen minutes. Fruits ordinarily take fifteen to twenty minutes to be prepared for absorption into your system; meats take about five hours to digest. However, when carbohydrates, starches and proteins are mixed, the stomach must quickly tailor its secretions to handle all types of food at one time. Forcing your stomach to process several different kinds of food all at once taxes your system. It's rather like trying to simultaneously balance your checkbook, calculate your income tax, and devise a budget. It can be done, but only inefficiently and with a lot of stress.

If you have a steak for dinner and cantaloup for dessert, you'll not be happy with the consequences. The sugar from the melon will be tied up along with the meat for about five hours. During that time the sugar will ferment and produce gas. The result is belching.

A fruit meal is digested very quickly. A high-protein breakfast of eggs, bacon, and toast, on the other hand, takes hours. You may be accustomed to a hearty breakfast that sees you through the first four or five hours of your day without major hunger pangs. You aren't hungry after the bacon and eggs breakfast because your body must work on it for so long. Your body is telling you, "Don't send anything else down here, I haven't finished cleaning up after the last mess." However, when you first institute an exclusively fruit breakfast, you may be hungry in about two hours. Despite the "hunger symptom," the fruit is doing better things for your body than the heavier breakfast.

Cantaloup and other melons eaten alone stay in the stomach for only about fifteen minutes, pass into the intestine, are assimilated, and turned into energy your body can use.

A meal of fruit is the ideal way to break your fast each day after sleeping. Fruit is so easily digested that it provides more energy than it uses in the digestive process. In addition, it encourages internal cleansing that helps rid your body of toxins.

Your protein meal should be the last meal of the day. Protein is a negative energy food. It takes more energy to process it than the protein provides. Give your body a chance to work on the protein during the period when you are least active and your energies can be directed toward digestion and assimilation.

To be sure, nearly all whole foods contain at least some protein, some carbohydrate, and some fat. We generally think of vegetables and fruits as being strictly carbohydrate: watermelon, for instance, with its 27 grams of carbohydrate in a 4" x 8" wedge. We don't ordinarily think of watermelon as containing fat and protein, but indeed it does. Not very much—about 2 grams of protein and 1 gram of fat.[1] By contrast, one-half of a 10-ounce avocado has 2 grams of protein and 18 grams of fat and only 6 grams of carbohydrate.[2]

Nearly all whole foods contain some carbohydrate, protein, and fat. In whole foods, carbohydrate, protein, or fat generally dominates according to volume. There will be a greater amount of one constituent than the others. The stomach works on the dominant constituent first, then goes to the next dominant type. The pH of the stomach is different when it is working on carbohydrates than when it is working on proteins. This is why it is so important to combine the foods you eat properly.

WELLNESS PRINCIPLE: *As we get older and/or sicker, food combining takes on greater importance.*

The food-combining chart and the list giving examples of foods in different food combining groups on the following pages can serve as a guide to follow in planning your meals. I don't recommend that all of the foods on the list be a part of your diet; but if they are, at least combine them in the way most advantageous to you.

The key to the chart is the single and double lines that separate the different groups of foods. Groups of foods that are separated by only a single line can be served at the same meal. For instance, starch foods and vegetables-salad; and protein and vegetables-salad. Sweet fruit and melons should not be combined with other foods. Allow an hour after eating fruit before eating another category of food.

FOOD - COMBINING CHART

SWEET FRUIT

STARCH

DAIRY

VEGETABLES SALAD

MELON

TART FRUIT

MEAT, NUTS

Generally, a food in the outer ring may be eaten with any food separated from it by only one line. For example, meat and nuts may be eaten with vegetables and salad, but not with starches or dairy.

Vegetables can be eaten with any of the acceptable combinations. Melons, sweet fruits, and tart fruits should be eaten alone.

FOOD-COMBINING GROUPS

SWEET FRUIT
Dried Figs
Dried Dates
Bananas
Raisins
Prunes
Avocado

DAIRY
Yogurt
Eggs (See Protein)
Milk
Cheese
Butter
Ice Cream

TART FRUIT - Acid
Limes
Sour Cherries
Tangerines
Strawberries
Grapefruit
Lemons
Pineapple
Oranges
Grapes
Plums
Cranberries

TART FRUIT -
Semi-Acid
Apricots
Blackberries
Peaches
Raspberries
Pears
Blueberries
Apples

MELONS
Cantaloup
Watermelon
Honeydew

VEGETABLES - SALADS
Spinach
Beet Greens
Celery
Chard Leaves
Watercress
Sauerkraut
Lettuce
Green Lima Beans
Cucumbers
Radishes
Rhubarb
Cabbage
Broccoli
Beets
Brussels Sprouts
Carrots
Green Soy Beans
Parsnips
Rutabagas
Cauliflower
Mushrooms
Green Beans
Onions
Green Peas
Fresh Corn
Tomatoes

STARCH

Molasses
Brown Sugar
Dried Beans
Dried Limas
White Potatoes
Ice Cream
Cookies
Corn Syrup
Granulated Sugar
Corn Oil
Olive Oil
Honey
Fresh Corn
Whole Wheat Bread
Barley, Pearled

Chocolate Cake
White Flour
Whole Wheat Flour
Brown Rice
White Bread
Macaroni
Spaghetti
Peanuts
Peanut Butter
Oatmeal
Soda Crackers
Dried Lentils
Wheat Germ
Wheat Bran
Oat Bran

PROTEIN
Pork
Lamb
Turkey
Beef
Veal
Chicken
Corned Beef
Bacon
Sausage

Shrimp
Salmon
Cod
Haddock
Sardines
Oysters
Scallops
Crab
Tuna
Whiting
Swordfish
Red Snapper

Dried Beans
Dried Lima
Dried Soy Beans
Dried Peas
Dried Lentils

Almonds
Brazil Nuts
Peanuts
Walnuts
Peanut Butter
Cashews
Macadamia Nuts
Filberts
Sunflower Seeds

Some general food-combining pointers to keep in mind:

- Protein and starches require completely different digestive environments. They should not be eaten together. (So much for a steak and baked potato, hamburger on a bun, or bagel and creamed cheese.)

- Protein should never be eaten with sweet fruit.

- Protein and sugar is one of the worst combinations (ice cream).

- Starches and fruits should not be eaten together (strawberry shortcake).

- Melons should be eaten alone—never in combination with other food.

- Begin each meal with something raw to allow the body to start manufacturing enzymes that can be carried over and used to produce your own enzymes.

- Fruit is the ideal food for the first meal of the day.

- A protein meal should be your last meal of the day.

- Liquids, including water, dilute digestive fluids; they should not be consumed with meals. Thirst doesn't accompany well-combined meals.

- Milk is not recommended. If you must drink milk, goat's milk is preferable to cow's milk.

WELLNESS PRINCIPLE: *Homemade ice cream is one of the best tasting, worst foods.*

GUIDELINES FOR HEALTHFUL MEALS

You may recall that in an earlier chapter of this book I recounted my clinical experiences that led to my investigations of the association between diet and health. I had observed that some patients responded to treatment more quickly than others. When it began to be clear to me that diet may play an important part in improvement time, I began asking quick-response and slow-response patients about their eating habits. I, like many others, "knew" that those patients who followed the tried-and-true Standard American Diet of three square meals a day were the ones who were responding faster. Surprisingly, I found the "junk food" gang responded faster than the "square mealers."

We have seen throughout this book how excess protein can impoverish the alkaline reserve of even the most well-intentioned health-seeker. A few sample menus should help to illustrate how we can innocently set ourselves up for disease. For example, a robust All American Breakfast can give us much more than we bargained for.

Breakfast

[1] 2 eggs   12 grams protein
    2 strips of bacon   4 grams protein
    hash browns   3 grams protein
    2 slices whole wheat bread   6 grams protein
    8 ounces orange juice   2 grams protein

When we put together all of these ingredients of a morning banquet, they spell Trouble with a capital T. This wonderfully nutritious breakfast has a grand total of 27 grams of protein, 22 of which come from acid ash-producing foods. That's 81% of the meal leaving acid ash. The hash browns and 8 ounces of orange juice will contribute alkaline ash and organic minerals to help neutralize some of the protein; however, this is about as effective as trying to sop up a glass of spilled milk with a Q-tip. Perhaps a lighter breakfast of cereal-and-coffee is better. Let's look:

[2] corn flakes with sugar   2 grams protein
    4 ounces milk   4 grams protein
    orange juice   2 grams protein
    coffee   0 protein and 0 nutrition

This less filling meal is probably more appropriate for those with a relatively sedentary lifestyle. And, interestingly, it is also less harmful to overall health than the heartier breakfast by virtue of the smaller amount of protein. Cereal, milk, and juice inflict a total of only 8 grams of protein as opposed to the 27 of the bacon and eggs menu. Granted, the cereal and milk are acid producers, but there is less protein as a whole. Again, the orange juice provides organic minerals for the alkaline reserve, and any acid produced as the o.j. is processed can be eliminated through the lungs.

On the other hand, let's look at what the hard-charging, I-don't-have-time-for-breakfast bunch gets when they gulp down a cup of coffee and a donut on the run.

| [3] 1 glazed donut | 3 grams protein |
| coffee | 0 protein—acid through and through |

No meat, little dairy, but all acid ash producers. This obviously "un-nutritious" meal wins the one-upmanship award over the hearty-breakfast-eaters menu—there isn't as much protein for the body to contend with. The donut, although made with acid ash-producing grains and covered with acid-generating sugar, has the advantage of being low in protein. It may not provide any additional ammunition for the alkaline reserve, but it doesn't greatly reduce the supply either. Some of the acid that is produced from this "junk food" breakfast can be eliminated through the lungs.

By contrast, the type breakfast recommended for those who prefer to feed their health as well as their appetites is not only light, appealing, and nutritious, but it also re-stocks vital organic minerals. A sample breakfast menu for those on the fast-track to health:

[4] 1 Banana	1 gram protein
1 Apple, sweet	0.2 grams protein
1 Pear, sweet	1 gram protein

This lively threesome not only restocks minerals, it introduces enzymes that help in their digestion. Fruit is "live" food. Our live bodies need live food to keep the energy flowing and in steady supply.

Just for purposes of comparison, a couple of midday and evening meal menus will illustrate beneficial and not-so-beneficial meals.

Mid-day Meal

[1] Hamburger on bun, lettuce
    and tomato   26 grams protein
   French fries (20 pieces)   4 grams protein
   Soft drink   0 grams protein
   85% acid ash-producing food plus acid-generating drink

[2] Fruit salad (1 cup)   1 gram protein
   Potato salad (1 cup)   7 grams protein
   Rye crackers (2 wafers)   2 grams protein
   80% alkaline ash-producing, 20% acid ash-producing; organic
   minerals available to replenish alkaline reserve

[3] Vegetable salad (lettuce, celery,
    green pepper, mushrooms,
    tomatoes, raw carrots,
    cucumber) (2 cups)   2 grams protein
   Whole wheat bread (1 slice) 3 gram protein
   100% alkaline ash-producing, and the alkaline reserve breathes a
   sigh of satisfaction

Evening Meal

[1] Steak (3 ounces)   20 grams protein
   Baked potato (1/2 lb)   4 grams protein
   Corn on the cob (1 ear)   4 grams protein
   Green beans (1/2 cup)   1 gram protein
   Coffee   0 grams protein
   82% acid ash-producing food plus acid-generating coffee. This is
   a standard "hearty dinner" for many households.

On a considerably less lavish scale, thousands of households squeeze a quick evening meal into their busy schedules of work, school, ball games for the children, community activities, and social commitments. A quick-fix meal, scarfed down in the interest of time might be:

[2] Cheese Pizza (3 slices)   18 grams protein
    Soft drink   0 grams protein
This quickie dumps 18 grams of protein plus a zero-nutrition, acid generating, acid containing soft drink.

An ideal evening meal is one that does your body the most good while it boosts your alkaline reserve.

[3] Vegetable salad (romaine,
      broccoli, cauliflower, onions,
      grated carrots, red cabbage,
      mushrooms) (1 cup)   1 gram protein
    Summer squash (1 cup)   2 grams protein
    Brown rice (1/2 cup cooked)   2.44 grams protein
Enough protein to keep your body functioning well, replenishing cells and staying in good repair without the burden of excess protein.

Your body was designed to sustain itself on food grown in nature— food that has been conditioned through the plant kingdom. Even so, there is nothing wrong with occasionally eating high-protein foods such as steak, Bar-B-Que, pizza, raw fish, chicken, pork chops and the like, as long as these foods don't make up the bulk of your diet. I do not advocate foregoing for all time your favorite foods and beverages. Your body can handle a limited amount of just about anything (short of poison) you care to give it. The secret is to give it predominantly the foods it needs to keep you healthy. Eating is a part of life; eating isn't all there is to life.

You don't need to make a fetish out of healthful eating. Once again, if you decide to treat yourself to a piece of eight-layer chocolate cake, enjoy it. In a future book I'll tell you how you can do as much damage to your physical body by carrying around guilt about your diet as you can by carrying around excess protein. Eat health-promoting foods *most* of the time.

Work into your new way of eating gradually. Changing the way you eat quickly is counterproductive to feeling good, even though, in the long run, it is good for your health. It is important that you feel comfortable with what you are doing. If you are unaccustomed to some of the foods that are health producers, prepare them in a way that is compatible with your current eating habits. As your health improves, your taste preferences will gravitate to those things your body needs.

If you aren't a breakfast eater, there's no need to begin now. Eat when you are hungry, not when the clock says it is time. After you are into the program and can eat generous quantities of fruit without suffering "digestive distress," have fruit for your first meal of the day.

Rigidity and fanaticism where eating is concerned are equally as detrimental to your health as faulty food. Begin adjusting your diet by modifying your current way of eating. We all have built-in psychological resistance to major changes of any well-established habit. Your first step is the Modified Diet.

Modified Diet

Include in Your Daily Diet: One serving of vegetables
                               One serving of fruit

When you are comfortable having additional vegetables and fruit, you can move into the Transitional Diet.

Transitional Diet

Transition: Increase amount of vegetables
                                  and fruit eaten each day
                               Have only vegetables for one meal
                                  each day
                               Increase number of fruit servings

If you have made the commitment to become as healthy as you can, your dietary goal is the Ideal Diet. However, even at the Transitional Diet stage, your health will be considerably better than you thought it could be. As your health improves, you will naturally gravitate toward better eating, without making a concerted effort. The Ideal Diet is a natural progression on the road to health. You will know when you are ready. Remember, your health is your choice.

Ideal Diet

Ideal Eating Pattern: Fruits and vegetables make
                               up 75% of your diet
                               Of the 75%, 30% is raw food
                               Grains, nuts, seeds, meat, fish, and
                               poultry make up the other 25% of
                               your diet
                               Processed, synthetic, or stimulatory
                               substances have been eliminated
                               from your diet

As a rule of thumb, breakfast should be a meal of fruit, the midday meal should be a starch meal, and the evening meal should be a protein meal.

The following examples can serve as a guide for meal planning. Remember, try to keep your protein consumption in the neighborhood of 25 grams per day.

Fruit Meals

1. Orange and grapefruit
2. Orange and pineapple
3. Grapefruit and sour apples
4. Bananas, pears, dates, sweet grapes
5. Figs, dates, sweet grapes, sweet apples

Starch Meals

1. Vegetable salad, carrots, potatoes, beets
2. Vegetable salad, asparagus, brown rice, cauliflower
3. Vegetable salad, green squash, fresh corn, asparagus
4. Vegetable salad, squash, okra, whole grain bread
5. Vegetable salad, broccoli, chard, kale, sweet potatoes

Protein Meals

1. Vegetable salad, green squash, spinach, nuts
2. Vegetable salad, yellow squash, cabbage, sunflower seeds
3. Vegetable salad, green beans, kale, cottage cheese
4. Vegetable salad, turnip greens, broccoli, eggs
5. Vegetable salad, baked potato, green beans, roast
   beef/chicken/turkey

Vegetable salad is a combination of any non-starch vegetables.

Let's put some of these meals together to see how the protein count adds up for one day.

Breakfast (Fruit Meal)	Grams Protein
Banana (1)	1
Pear (1)	1
White grapes (5.5 oz)	1.6
Apple (1) .	2
Total grams protein	3.8

Midday Meal (Starch Meal)	
Vegetable salad* (1 cup)	±2.5
Squash, summer (1/2 cup)	1
Kale (1/2 cup)	2
Whole wheat bread (1 slice)	3
Total grams protein	8.5

Evening Meal (Protein Meal)	
Vegetable salad* (1 cup)	±2.5
Asparagus (1/2 cup)	3
Baked potato	4
Egg (1)	6
Total grams protein	15.5
Total protein for the day	27.8

* Vegetable salad of red cabbage, green beans, cauliflower, broccoli, beets, and mushrooms

You can see that it doesn't take much for the protein total to mount up. Just by adding another egg (6 grams), you can take the total to 33.8 grams a day. If you substitute a 3-ounce piece of roast beef for the eggs, the protein total for the day zooms up to 38 grams.

However, on the good news side, even if you add yet another 2 grams of protein by putting macaroni and red kidney beans in your evening vegetable salad, your alkaline-ash/acid-ash ratio for the day is quite favorable. Remember, it's proportions that make the difference. Instead of your diet being made up of 80% or more of acid ash-producing foods, work toward having your daily menus made up of 75% or more alkaline ash-producing foods.

The sample menus shown here can serve as a guide as you begin your journey to health through diet. Even though some of the combinations may not be perfect, it's a beginning. As time goes on, you will create your own menus to suit your own tastes. Your goal is to reach proportions of 75% alkaline ash and 25% acid ash foods. The foods you choose as you move in that direction are up to you. Only you can keep your internal environment in top form by giving it the best fuel you can.

CHAPTER 23

Exercise–The Cherry on Top

A book about getting and staying healthy wouldn't be complete without a few words about exercise. My earlier analogy of the body as a well-tuned engine that needs the proper fuel to run can be carried a step farther. Just as you can't expect a carefully synchronized engine to run well on inferior fuel, you can't expect that precision machine to function at its best if it is never allowed to operate at full capacity. Parts can suffer from lack of use. In the same vein, our parts need exercise. Unfortunately, not everyone is healthy enough to exercise their veins vigorously.

Throughout this book I have cautioned against engaging in strenuous exercise if your urine pH is very high in the morning after you have eaten an acid ash meal. The purpose of this repeated caution is not to instill fear and apprehension in weekend athletes but to help you to understand that you need to be healthy before you push your body too far. Just how far is "too far" depends upon where you start.

Exercise can be disastrous if your body is already over-stressed by acid. Acid generated by physical exertion is added to an already high acid level. The internal environment can become so acid that the heart cannot continue to function. Although this hypothesis has not been "proved" by hard quantitative data, consider the high incidence of young athletes in apparently "good health" who succumb unexpectedly to cardiac arrest or heart attacks during or following strenuous exercise.

Reports appear regularly in sports periodicals announcing the death of apparently "healthy" athletes: a twenty-year old collegiate football player dies while playing summer basketball in gym; a football coach succumbs to a heart attack at age forty-eight after working out; a former university basketball player, age twenty-eight, dies after jogging; a twenty-year old college football player dies of cardiac arrest after a "conditioning session." Being fit isn't the same as being healthy.

You don't get healthy by exercising. You get healthy by giving your body the kind of food that allows it to maintain the steady-state of homeostasis and to function effortlessly. Until your pH readings show that your body is in the alkaline range, your exercise sessions shouldn't raise your heart rate above 120 beats per minute. If your morning urine pH readings are between 6.8 and 7.4 after an alkaline ash meal the night before, or if your morning pH is 5.8 or below after an acid ash meal, your body can handle the additional acid generated by strenuous exercise. You can work on becoming more fit. If you can't claim this level of health, work on your diet before you exercise.

WELLNESS PRINCIPLE: *Health is served at the meal table; muscles and stamina are built by exercise.*

Most of the more popular forms of exercise are aerobic—sustained activities that cause you to breathe deeply and to take more oxygen than usual into your lungs. Running, jogging, walking, tennis, aerobic dancing, and the like are intensive activities performed continuously for blocks of time, usually twenty minutes to several hours. All of these aerobic exercises can benefit your heart-lung complex. Weight lifting and simple gardening are anaerobic activities that can increase muscle strength but fall short of sustaining increased heart or breathing rates. Anaerobic exercise involves short bursts of muscular activity that may increase the rate of your pulse and breathing intermittently for only brief periods.

Football, boxing, bull-fighting, automobile racing, and giant slalom skiing all require strength, stamina, and coordination; however, much of the appeal of these potentially dangerous sports seems to be more from the stimulation involved with the thrill of risk-taking than from a burning desire to improve health. Beneficial exercise programs they aren't. They are activities that require other exercise as preparation—training. The training is more beneficial to health than participating in the sport itself.

When done correctly, exercise can be the cherry on top of a healthful way of eating. Unfortunately, not all exercise is good for you. Injuries result when you put undue strain on muscles, joints, or your internal communication system. Frequently, the conditions under which the exercise is performed reduce its intrinsic benefits: running on hard surfaces for long distances; exercising in extreme heat or cold; over-exercising that stresses both mind and body. Excessive exercising or exercising at inappropriate times can turn benefits into liabilities.

Some sports and activities are more beneficial than others to the well-being of both your neurological system and your cardiovascular system. These are the sports that involve contralateral movement: alternating simultaneous movement of the right arm and left leg with the left arm and right leg. Basketball, soccer, running, swimming crawl or backstroke all require alternating right and left movements of opposite arms and legs. On the other hand, tennis, golf, and baseball are "one-sided" sports—the swing is always to the same side. The saving grace for these is that they also require running or walking. If you ride a cart when you play golf, you aren't getting the most benefit from the game, even though you may do a lot of arm-swinging if you are a high-handicapper.

WELLNESS PRINCIPLE: *Golf is good exercise only if you walk from tee to green.*

Weight lifting and bicycle riding are not contralateral exercises. Weight lifting involves using arms and legs in unison during short bursts of strenuous activity. Bicycling gives the legs and cardiovascular system a good workout, but the arms and upper body may remain relatively static. Although both weight lifting and bicycle riding can be beneficial in their own ways, they should be followed immediately by a period of contralateral walking that includes swinging the arms.

Some stationary exercise bicycles do provide contralateral bene-fits. These are the exercise bicycles with handlebars that move alter-nately as the pedals rotate. The right handle bar moves toward the body while the left moves away, then they reverse the pattern. Sur-prisingly, there is a "right" way and a "wrong" way to use these, as one of my clinic staff members discovered. She had bought a classy exer-cise bike and began using it. She soon noticed that each time she "rode" her bike, she developed a headache. This physiological re-sponse just wasn't logical. She was getting good exercise with a con-tralateral pattern that should have eliminated headaches, not induced them. We analyzed what she was doing and found that she was pulling on the handlebars. When she altered the pattern and *pushed* on each handlebar, she didn't develop a headache.

In her original pattern, she was, in effect, exercising homolater-ally. She was stressing her right leg by pushing down on the pedal and her right arm by pulling on the handlebar, then repeating the proce-dure with her left leg and left arm. She wasn't getting the benefit of contralateral movement. This incident illustrates that the way you ex-ercise can mean the difference between pain and pleasure.

Therapeutic exercise strengthens muscles, improves the cardio-vascular system, increases energy, increases bone density, and, when combined with proper dietary habits, may help in weight control. As with improving health, losing weight begins at the meal table. Exer-cise, however, is an adjunct to proper eating that can assist in weight control. But don't expect exercise to take off pounds if too much of the wrong kind of food is going into your mouth.

One of benefits of exercise that is difficult to measure is the in-crease in your mental feeling of well-being. Even moderate exercise such as walking, dancing, gardening, and low-impact aerobics stimu-lates endorphin production. Endorphins are chemical substances produced in the brain that boost your spirits and act as pain killers or analgesics. The more consistently you exercise, the more consistently endorphins are produced and the better you feel.

Walking is probably the best exercise for the greatest number of people. Everyone who can get up and move around can benefit from a program of proper walking. However, there is a right way and a wrong way to walk.

Walking is an invigorating exercise that stimulates but doesn't stress the body's natural rhythms. When done properly, walking is excellent contralateral action. Your arms should be allowed to swing freely at your sides; walking balances your internal systems best when you aren't resting your hands in your pockets or carrying something. When your arms swing freely at your sides, the internal communication that keeps your body functioning properly improves. As your right arm swings forward when you step out with your left foot (and vice versa), your arms act as a natural balancing device for your neurological and physiological systems.

Brisk walking relaxes and tones the lower back muscles that are associated with the diaphragm. As a result, walking helps relieve the symptoms of a hiatus hernia. Walking also promotes proper function of the lungs, stomach, cardiovascular, and elimination systems. To top it all off, contralateral walking improves blood circulation and stimulates transportation of oxygen to all parts of the body including the brain. A regular program of walking can help the symptoms of headache sufferers. There's a lot to be said for walking when it's done right.

You should wear loose-fitting clothing that is appropriate for the weather; and correctly fitting, comfortable shoes. Leave your cassette player with headphones at home when you walk. Walking benefits are reduced dramatically when intrusive sounds are forced on the brain.

Take comfortable-length strides. Don't shorten or lengthen your stride to match that of another person's. Walk tall. Be relaxed. Hold your head high. Keep your shoulders back and your back straight.

If you haven't been getting much exercise, begin therapeutic walking slowly and increase your speed and distance gradually to suit your own level of stamina. You should walk just fast enough to increase your pulse rate to about 120 beats per minute. This provides the positive aerobic effects of running or jogging without putting undue strain on your cardiovascular system, legs, knees, ankles, or feet.

Walking upright with contralateral movement is a natural progression from the cross-crawl motion we learn as infants. Babies who are confined to playpens often skip the crawling stage and go directly to walking. Early-age walking may be gratifying to parents who are impressed by their child's obvious genius and outstanding coordination, but the child misses a vital part of his neurological development process. Similarly, infants who are put in walkers to encourage walking at an early age are deprived of natural developmental crawling exercise.

We develop neurologically in stages. In early infancy, same-side arm and leg movements originate in the lower centers of the brain, primarily the pons. At about six months, the contralateral cross-crawl patterns originating in the mid-brain area begin to become more evident. The child is on his way to becoming an upright citizen. Walking involves the development of ever higher centers of the brain.

We take a long time to perfect our contralateral movements. As toddlers, wobbling about the house takes concentration. Months of practice are needed before fast wobbling evolves into one-foot-in-front-of-the-other walking, and finally to the true both-feet-off- the-floor springing action of running.

As we move into old age, contralateral patterns seem to diminish. Debilitating illness and feelings of tentative balance lead to a shuffling gait. Shuffling is not therapeutic walking. It is a means of upright locomotion, but the neurological benefits of contralateral movement are missing. I had an elderly neighbor who used to "walk" almost every morning. She moved from one location to another all right, however, her feet never left the ground and her arms were held woodenly at her sides. She wasn't getting nearly as much benefit from her daily constitutional as she imagined. Had she at least swung her arms contralaterally with her stride, her exercise sessions would have been more beneficial. She would have felt better and been able to walk more confidently.

Keep the contralateral concept in mind. The next time you have a headache or muscle ache, try "walking" it out. Make sure that you walk properly, however. Swing those arms, and step out with confidence and natural ease.

Exercise can help you have more energy, move more easily, and feel better. Health is a whole-body condition. To get (or stay) in top form, you need to use your body to the best of its abilities and fuel it with the food that is best for it.

WELLNESS PRINCIPLE: *Health is dished up at meals—exercise is the cherry on top.*

Epilogue

You now have some fundamentals about

- how your body works to keep you alive,
- how to monitor your current level of health,
- how food in general causes responses in your body,
- how too much protein leads to chronic degenerative disease,
- the importance of keeping your body slightly alkaline,
- meal planning,
- food combining,
- proper exercise, and
- your choice of health.

Now let's talk Real World.

Interest in health improvement is on the rise; smoking is no longer socially acceptable, and lowering cholesterol is "in." Many of the people who attend the Concentrated Care Program at Morter Clinic are interested in *improving* their health; they are not seriously ill. They participate in these four-day programs because they want to be even healthier, happier, and more successful; they are committed to health.

Yet in our society, the chances of most of us following unswervingly the guidelines I have set down in this book are almost as good as those of successfully stacking marbles. We live in a social setting: families, friends, business associates, civic organizations, church and synagog groups. We eat together. Even if you commit to never violating any of the principles set forth in this book, you may find little, if any, support from family and associates. Family and friends sometimes feel "threatened" when we try to improve ourselves. Those who diverge from traditional eating patterns are often viewed as "food freaks." Street-wise pseudo sophisticates do not smile on others whose practices appear to set a standard of self-discipline higher than their own. To compound the problem, our tastes are so ingrained that we blanch at the prospect of "giving up" our tried and true food favorites.

I am not suggesting that you never eat your favorite foods again. I am simply encouraging you to be aware of how your body must respond to the substances you put into it. I have given you concepts of how to feed your body so that you will get the most mileage from it most comfortably. Any improvement in your diet will improve your health. Take your time. Go at your own pace. Set your own goals. It's your life and your level of comfort. It's your health and your choice.

At least now you have a base from which to guide your own health life. You are the one who can make the choice as to how healthy you want to be.

A patient at our clinic who had suffered from a form of arthritis for about eight years dramatically altered his eating pattern. He entered his new dietary program quite skeptically. After all, even the authorities on arthritis denied that food has anything to do with this painful, debilitating disease. Their attitude was that food has little bearing on arthritis and that the best diet plan is to eat balanced meals. "Balanced" includes the four basic food groups we have grown up with.

For over ten years now, this fellow has been following his "new" way of eating. There may be a way to knock him off of his routine (threaten his children or grandchildren); but almost nothing would induce him to return to his pain-producing former way of eating.

He was diligent and conscientious in following his program, and improvement in his case was obvious within a week. Yet he met with an amazing response from friends and acquaintances who observed his progress. "You look so much better," many remarked. "I have arthritis in my hands/knees/shoulders. What did you do?" After he had given them a thumb-nail sketch of his diet program, almost every one of these "arthritis sufferers" retorted that they couldn't "give up" cheese, or meat, or some other favorite. His reply to their protestations was, "Then you don't hurt bad enough yet."

You may "hurt bad enough," or you may be tired of being tired. Or you may just be ready to live the rest of your life feeling better than you do now. If you decide to eat for better health, whatever your reason, it's *your* reason. Sickness is not a natural by-product of life. And you don't have to be sick in order to want to feel better. If you want to feel better, you now have the tools. It's up to you. You don't have to develop cancer or AIDS to become motivated to eat a better diet.

You make the choice as to how you respond to the temptation of eating favorite foods that affect you unfavorably. You can choose to eat them and pay the price of the reaction you have; you can decline to eat them by going with the current trend of claiming a "sensitivity" to those foods; or you can improve your dietary habits in general so that your overall invisible health improves. If you elect the last choice, your body will be able to handle your daily diet without adverse reactions, and it will cope with occasional flings, with barely a symptomatic ripple.

No matter what your decision, make it and be comfortable with it. You can always change later if you choose to. The most important thing is that you don't feel guilty about the things you eat. You are better off eating things that are "bad" for you and feeling good about it than eating things that are "good" for you and feeling bad about it. You do more damage to your body by the way you think than by eating the wrong kinds of food. But that's the next book.

Endnotes

CHAPTER 5

1. Guyton, Arthur C., M.D., *Textbook of Medical Physiology*, 7th Edition. (Philadelphia: W.B. Saunders Co., 1986), p. 277

CHAPTER 8

1. Guyton, Arthur C., M.D., *Textbook of Medical Physiology*, 7th Edition. (Philadelphia: W.B. Saunders Co., 1986), p. 438
2. Hodgman, Charles D., M.S., Robert C. Weast, Ph.D., Samuel M. Selby, Ph.D., *Handbook of Chemistry and Physics*, 40th ed. (Cleveland: Chemical Rubber Publishing Co., 1958), p. 1721
3. Cantarow, Abraham, M.D., Bernard Schepartz, Ph.D., *Biochemistry*. (Philadelphia and London: W.B. Saunders Company, 1954), pp. 261, 262, 267
4. Guyton, p. 772

CHAPTER 9

1. Guyton, Arthur C., M.D., *Textbook of Medical Physiology*, 7th Edition. (Philadelphia: W.B. Saunders Co., 1986), p. 790
2. Cantarow, Abraham, M.D., Bernard Schepartz, Ph.D., *Biochemistry*. (Philadelphia and London: W.B. Saunders Company, 1954), p. 262
3. Guyton, p. 780
4. *Taber's Cyclopedic Medical Dictionary*, Edition 15, Clayton L. Thomas, M.D., M.P.H., ed. (Philadelphia: F.A. David Co., 1958), p. 526

5. Orten, James M., Ph.D., and Otto W. Neuhaus, Ph.D., *Human Bio-chemistry*. (Saint Louis: The C.V. Mosby Company, 1975), p. 464
6. Taber's, p. 657

CHAPTER 10
1. *Taber's Cyclopedic Medical Dictionary*, Edition 15, Clayton L. Thomas, M.D., M.P.H., ed. (Philadelphia: F.A. David Co., 1958), p. 141
2. "How's Your Lunch?," *Hippocrates*, 3:1, January/February 1989, p. 57
3. *1990 Medical and Health Annual*, Philip W. Goetz, Editor in Chief. (Chicago: Encyclopaedia Britannica, Inc., 1989), pp. 21-23
4. Orten, James M., Ph.D., and Otto W. Neuhaus, Ph.D., *Human Bio-chemistry*. (Saint Louis: The C.V. Mosby Company, 1975), p. 627
5. Robinson, Corinne, H., *Proudfit-Robinson's Normal and Therapeutic Nutrition*, 13th ed. (London: The Macmillan Company, Collier-Macmillan Limited, 1967), p. 657
6. Richardson, Dr. R.A., *Increasing the Strength of the Eyes and the Eye Muscles Without the Aid of Glasses*. (Kansas City, MO: The Eyesight and Health Association Publishers, 1926), pp. 164-166

CHAPTER 13
1. Guyton, Arthur C., M.D., *Textbook of Medical Physiology*, 7th Edition. (Philadelphia: W.B. Saunders Co., 1986), p. 7
2. Guyton, pp. 14-15
3. Orten, James M., Ph.D., and Otto W. Neuhaus, Ph.D., *Human Bio-chemistry*. (Saint Louis: The C.V. Mosby Company, 1975), p. 253
4. Guyton, p. 12
5. Guyton, p. 48
6. Guyton, p. 35

CHAPTER 14
1. Guyton, Arthur C., M.D., *Textbook of Medical Physiology*, 7th Edition. (Philadelphia: W.B. Saunders Co., 1986), p. 829
2. Orten, James M., Ph.D., and Otto W. Neuhaus, Ph.D., *Human Bio-chemistry*. (Saint Louis: The C.V. Mosby Company, 1975), p. 716

3. Morter, M.T., Jr., D.C. *Correlative Urinalysis*. (Rogers, AR: B.E.S.T. Research, Inc., 1987), p. 82
4. Orten & Neuhaus, p. 710
5. Guyton, p. 862
6. McDougall, John A., M.D., and Mary A. McDougall, *The McDougall Plan*. (Piscataway, N.J.: New Century Publishers, 1983), p. 95
7. McDougall, p. 101
8. Orten & Neuhaus, p. 690
9. Anand, Chander Rekha, and Hellen M. Linkswiler, "Effect of Protein Intake on Calcium Balance of Young Men Given 500 mg Calcium Daily," *Journal of Nutrition* 104:695-700, 1974, p. 698
10. Guyton, p. 790
11. Nutrition Action Health Letter, 14:2, March 1987, p. 4

CHAPTER 15

1. Cantarow, Abraham, M.D., Bernard Schepartz, Ph.D., *Biochemistry*. (Philadelphia and London: W.B. Saunders Company, 1954), pp. 260-261
2. Guyton, Arthur C., M.D., *Textbook of Medical Physiology*, 7th Edition. (Philadelphia: W.B. Saunders Co., 1986), p. 444
3. Guyton, p. 484
4. Tuttle, W.W., Ph.D., Sc.D., and Byron A. Schottelius, Ph.D., *Textbook of Physiology*, 14th ed. (St. Louis: The C.V. Mosby Company, 1961), pp. 389-390

CHAPTER 16

1. Bieler, Henry G., M.D., *Food is Your Best Medicine*. (New York: Random House, Vintage Books Division, 1973), p. 190
2. Bieler, p. 196
3. Bieler, p. 192

CHAPTER 17

1. *Taber's Cyclopedic Medical Dictionary*, Edition 15, Clayton L. Thomas, M.D., M.P.H., ed. (Philadelphia: F.A. David Co., 1958), p. 2052
2. Orten, James M., Ph.D., and Otto W. Neuhaus, Ph.D., *Human Biochemistry*. (Saint Louis: The C.V. Mosby Company, 1975), p. 531

3. Manahan, William, M.D., *Eat for Health: A Do-It-Yourself Nutrition Guide for Solving Common Medical Problems.* (Tiburon, CA: H.J. Kramer, Inc., 1988), p. 48

4. Guyton, Arthur C., M.D., *Textbook of Medical Physiology*, 7th Edition. (Philadelphia: W.B. Saunders Co., 1986), pp. 261-262

5. Bieler, Henry G., M.D., *Food is Your Best Medicine.* (New York: Random House, Vintage Books Division, 1973), p. 219

6. Bieler, p. 219

7. Kurtz, T.W., M.D., Hamoudi A. Al-Bander, M.D., and R. Curtis Morris, Jr., M.D., "'Salt-Sensitive' Essential Hypertension in Men: Is the Sodium Ion Alone Important?," *New England Journal of Medicine*, Vol. 317, 17:1043-1048, 1987, p. 1045

8. Kurtz, et al, p. 1048

9. Guyton, p. 436

10. Kurtz, et al, p. 1048

11. *Reader's Digest*, Vol 133, No. 799, November 1988, pp. 17-22

12. Orten & Neuhaus, p. 713

13. Orten & Neuhaus, p. 531

CHAPTER 18

1. McDougall, John A., M.D., and Mary A. McDougall, *The McDougallPlan.* (Piscataway, N.J.: New Century Publishers, 1983), p. 102

2. Allen, Lindsay H., Ph.D., E.A. Oddoye, Ph.D., and S. Margen, M.D., "Protein-induced hypercalciuria: a longer term study," *The American Journal of Clinical Nutrition*, 32:741-749, April 1979, p. 741

3. Bieler, Henry G., M.D., *Food is Your Best Medicine.* (New York: Random House, Vintage Books Division, 1973), p. 213

4. Robinson, Corinne, H., *Proudfit-Robinson's Normal and Therapeutic Nutrition*, 13th ed. (London: The Macmillan Company, Collier-Macmillan Limited, 1967), p. 835

5. Kamen, Betty, Ph.D., and Si Kamen, *Osteoporosis: What It Is, How to Prevent It, How to Stop It.* (New York: Pinnacle Books, Inc., 1984), p. 146

CHAPTER 19
1. Arias, Irwin M., M.D., David Schachter, M.D., Hans Popper, M.D., David A. Shafritz, M.D., *The Liver Biology and Pathobiology*. (New York: Raven Press, 1982), p. 467
2. Guyton, Arthur C., M.D., *Textbook of Medical Physiology*, 7th Edition. (Philadelphia: W.B. Saunders Co., 1986), p. 825
3. University of California, Berkeley Wellness Letter, Rodney M. Friedman, Editor and Publisher, March 1989, Vol. 5, Issue 6, pp. 4-5
4. University of California, Berkeley Wellness Letter, p. 6
5. "New Cholesterol Clue," *Hippocrates*, 3:3, May/June 1989, pp. 16, 18

CHAPTER 20
1. Bear, Firman E., Stephen J. Toth, and Arthur L. Prince, "Variation in Mineral Composition of Vegetables," *Soil Science Society Proceedings*, 1948, Vol. 13, pp. 380-384.
2. *Taber's Cyclopedic Medical Dictionary*, Edition 15, Clayton L. Thomas, M.D., M.P.H., ed. (Philadelphia: F.A. David Co., 1958), p. 68
3. Orten, James M., Ph.D., and Otto W. Neuhaus, Ph.D., *Human Biochemistry*. (Saint Louis: The C.V. Mosby Company, 1975), p. 522
4. Guyton, Arthur C., M.D., *Textbook of Medical Physiology*, 7th Edition. (Philadelphia: W.B. Saunders Co., 1986), p. 45
5. Guyton, p. 45
6. Sehnert, Keith W., M.D., *The Garden Within: Acidophilus - Candida Connection*. (Burlingame, CA: Health World, Inc., 1989), p. 5
7. Guyton, p. 861
8. Guyton, p. 862

CHAPTER 22
1. Robinson, Corinne, H., *Proudfit-Robinson's Normal and Therapeutic Nutrition*, 13th ed. (London: The Macmillan Company, Collier-Macmillan Limited, 1967), p. 806
2. Robinson, p. 764

Index

heredity, 7
homeostasis, 109
hypothalamus, 114

infants, 87
inhibitors, health, 40, 204
inorganic, 58, 140
intelligence, internal, 118
internal environment, 26, 110
ion, 109, 123
irridiated food, 80, 205

Kreb's cycle, 112

Lemon Egg, 212
lemon test, 95, 104
lipoprotein(a), 178
liver, 68, 172, 187
    cell, 112, 115

margarine, 204
metabolic activity, 118
milk, 166
    cow, 166
    goat, 87
    human, 87, 125, 127, 166,
        183
    pasteruization, 166
minerals, 58, 140
    of alkaline reserve, 78
mitochondria, 112

Natural, Normal, Necessary, 21
nitrogen, 120
    ammonia, 121

organelles, 111
organic, 58, 140
osmotic balance, 117
osteoporosis, 59, 73, 137, 161—170
oxidation, 81, 83

pancreas, 67
pH, 53—56
    and exercise, 234
    extracellular, 55
    intracellular, 55
    of body fluids, 55
    of enzymes, 65—66
    test paper, 91
phosphorus, 167
plaque, 173, 177
potassium, 138, 150, 154
pregnancy, 79
protein, 117—129, 188
    complete, 129, 182
    content of foods, 127, 162, 196
    dietary, 118
    effects on calcium balance, 128
    energy, 118, 222
    excess, 3, 26, 110, 117, 126
    of cells, 109, 117
    percentage of diet, 1, 127
    requirements, 36, 120, 126, 129,
        189
    stimulation, 119

saliva, 65, 71, 74
    ph, 104
    testing, 94
salt, 74, 142, 147—160
sleep, 90, 106
sodium, 120, 135, 147—160
    bicarbonate, 155
    chloride, 155